Eat, Move, Thrive: The Female Blueprint

By

KIRAN VEKARIYA

ISBN:9798861499613

DEDICATION

To all females of the World…

CONTENTS

ACKNOWLEDGMENTS

Writing a book is a journey that rarely happens alone. It's a collaborative effort that draws from the support and inspiration of many. As I reflect on the creation of "Eat, Move, Thrive: The Female Blueprint," I am humbled and grateful for the incredible individuals who have contributed to its existence.

First and foremost, I would like to express my deepest gratitude to my family for their unwavering support and understanding throughout this journey. Your love and encouragement have been my pillars of strength.

To my dear friends and colleagues, your enthusiasm and belief in this project have been instrumental in its completion. Your valuable insights and feedback have enriched the content and made it more accessible to readers.

I extend my heartfelt thanks to the dedicated team who worked tirelessly behind the scenes to bring this book to life. Your expertise and commitment to excellence are reflected in every page.

I am deeply appreciative of the countless individuals who have shared their stories and experiences, adding authenticity and relatability to the content. Your openness to share your journeys has made this book more than just words on paper; it is a tapestry of real-life inspiration.

To the readers, I extend my warmest appreciation. Your curiosity and quest for knowledge have driven the creation of this book. It is my hope that the insights within these pages empower you on your own path to well-being.

Finally, I must acknowledge the unwavering support of the entire wellness community. Your dedication to improving the lives of others has inspired me throughout this process. Together, we are creating a healthier, happier world.

In every sense, this book is a collective endeavor, a shared vision of holistic well-being for women everywhere. It is with deep gratitude that I extend my thanks to each and every one of you. Your contributions have made "Eat, Move, Thrive" a reality, and for that, I am truly thankful.

With warm regards,

Kiran Vekariya.

FOREWORD

In my decades of research and consultations with women from all walks of life, I've come to recognize a universal truth: our bodies, minds, and spirits are intricately connected. The challenges and triumphs we experience in one facet of our lives reverberate through the others. Yet, mainstream discussions on health and wellness often silo these facets, rarely addressing them in tandem.

"Eat, Move, Thrive: The Female Blueprint" is my attempt to weave these threads together into a comprehensive guide for women. This book doesn't just discuss diets or exercise routines; it's a celebration of women's unique physiology and the incredible symphony of processes that occur within us.

From understanding the rhythmic dance of our hormonal cycles to the transformative journey of pregnancy and the empowering transition of menopause, this book serves as a compass. Each chapter is meticulously researched, drawing upon the latest scientific findings, age-old wisdom, and the personal stories of countless women I've had the honor of guiding over the years.

As you journey through these pages, my hope is that you'll discover not just the knowledge but also the tools and strategies to craft your own blueprint. A blueprint that respects your individuality, celebrates your strengths, and empowers you to thrive in every season of life.

Thank you for allowing me to be a part of your journey.
Here's to a life of vibrant health, boundless energy, and
unyielding spirit!

With gratitude and respect,

Kiran Vekariya

PREFACE

"Eat, Move, Thrive: The Female Blueprint" is a holistic approach to women's health. It recognizes that women have unique health needs due to factors like hormones, menstruation, and menopause.

When it comes to nutrition, women should focus on a balanced diet with plenty of fruits, vegetables, lean proteins, and whole grains. Staying hydrated is crucial, too.

Regular exercise is essential for women. It helps with weight management, cardiovascular health, and bone strength. Cardio workouts and strength training are both important.

Hormonal balance is key. Stress management, quality sleep, and avoiding excessive caffeine and alcohol can help. Some women may consider hormone replacement therapy during menopause, but it should be discussed with a healthcare provider.

Emotional health matters just as much as physical health. Mindfulness, counseling, and a good support network can make a big difference.

Don't forget preventive care. Regular check-ups, cancer screenings, and vaccinations are essential.

Lifestyle choices like not smoking and moderating alcohol intake can significantly impact health.

Remember, every woman is unique, so a personalized approach to health is important.

In a nutshell, "Eat, Move, Thrive: The Female Blueprint" provides a holistic framework for women's health, addressing physical, emotional, and lifestyle factors to help women thrive throughout their lives. Always consult with healthcare professionals for personalized guidance.

1 INTRODUCTION: CELEBRATING THE FEMALE FORM: UNPACKING THE UNIQUE ASPECTS OF WOMEN'S HEALTH

Hey there, beautiful soul!

Let's start by imagining we're in a serene spot, perhaps a cozy nook in a bustling café, the tantalizing aroma of fresh coffee wafting through the air. Or maybe, we're sitting on a sun-drenched porch, surrounded by the chirping of birds and a gentle breeze. Imagine us sharing stories, laughs, and those cherished "Aha!" moments. Now, with that delightful setting in mind, welcome to our shared journey into the intricate, awe-inspiring world of women's health.

Ah, women's health. It sounds so clinical, doesn't it? But trust me, by the end of this book, you're going to see it as a treasure trove of insights, mysteries, and stories that make up the incredible journey of being a woman. Let's kick things off with a heart-to-heart about the beauty, challenges, and sheer magic of the female form.

It's vital that we recognize and celebrate the unique aspects of women's health. One fundamental aspect is the reproductive system. Women experience menstruation, pregnancy, and menopause, each of which comes with its own set of health considerations.

Menstruation, for instance, involves hormonal fluctuations that can impact mood and physical comfort. It's essential for women to understand their menstrual cycle and how to manage any discomfort or irregularities.

Pregnancy is a transformative time for women's bodies. Proper prenatal care is crucial to ensure both maternal and fetal health. This includes regular check-ups, a balanced diet, and exercise tailored to the individual's needs.

Menopause marks another significant transition. Hormonal changes during this phase can lead to symptoms like hot flashes and mood swings. Women should explore options for managing these symptoms, which may include hormone replacement therapy or lifestyle adjustments.

Breast health is also unique to women. Regular breast self-exams and mammograms are essential for early detection of breast cancer. It's a practice that can literally save lives.

Bone health is another aspect that deserves attention. Women are more susceptible to osteoporosis, and a diet rich in calcium and vitamin D, along with weight-bearing exercises, can help maintain strong bones.

Mental health is a critical component of overall well-being. Women may face unique stressors related to societal expectations and roles. Strategies like therapy, meditation, or simply reaching out for support can make a big difference.

It's important to remember that women's health isn't just about reproductive and physical aspects. Emotional health, societal factors, and access to healthcare all play crucial roles. Celebrating the female form means embracing and addressing these multifaceted aspects of women's health.

An Ode to Our Unique Design

Isn't it fascinating how we, as women, are designed? Our bodies can nurture a new life, adapt to different life stages, and have this innate ability to connect deeply with others and with ourselves. The ebb and flow of our monthly cycles, the rich tapestry of emotions we can experience in just a day, the intricate balance of hormones that can either make us feel on top of the world or like we want to hide under the covers - these are all a part of our unique blueprint.

But here's a truth bomb: while society has evolved leaps and bounds, there's still a lot of mystery shrouding women's health. From the misconceptions about our monthly cycles to the one-size-fits-all approach to diets and fitness, we're often left navigating this journey with a map that, well, doesn't quite match our terrain.

Dismantling Myths, Building Connections

As we dive into this exploration, one of our foremost aims is to dismantle myths. Have you ever been told that mood swings are "just a part of being a woman" or that "women are just more emotional"? Well, we're here to break down such stereotypes, to decode the science behind these statements, and find out the truth.

Moreover, this journey isn't just about understanding our bodies. It's about building a deeper, more loving connection with ourselves. It's about listening intently to our body's whispers (or sometimes its loud cries for attention), and realizing that every sign, every symptom is its way of communicating with us.

The Spectrum of Women's Health

Before we get any further, let's be clear: women's health is not just about reproductive health. It's a spectrum, embracing everything from the physical to the emotional, from the cellular level to our overall well-being. It's about understanding our bodies, listening to them, and ensuring we provide them what they need at every stage of our lives.

Your Body, Your Story

Isn't it odd how from a young age we're taught about the world around us, about math, history, and science, but so little time is spent on teaching us about our own bodies? Especially, the unique aspects of the female body?

Take a moment and think back. Did anyone ever sit you down and explain the intricacies of your menstrual cycle? Or delve into the emotional roller coaster that hormones can sometimes be? Probably not, right? Most of us had to figure it out ourselves, often through trial and error.

Our bodies have been whispering their stories to us for ages. The mild acne breakout before our periods, the bloating, the mood swings, or the inexplicable energy surges. They all mean something. They're clues, guiding us to understand our deeper selves.

The Power of Intuition

You know that gut feeling you get sometimes? Call it intuition or a sixth sense; it's real, and it's powerful. Throughout history, women have been known to possess a unique intuitive ability. This intuition can often guide us in understanding our health, too. Have you ever felt 'off' without being able to pinpoint why? Or felt incredibly energetic and vibrant on some days without any particular reason? That's your intuition speaking.

As we journey through this book, one thing I'd love for you to do is to reignite and trust that intuition. Listen to your body. Sometimes, it might just be hinting at a larger narrative that's waiting to be unraveled.

Beyond The Stereotypes

A pivotal part of this journey will be to challenge and push beyond stereotypes. Women's health, unfortunately, has been plagued by a plethora of myths and misconceptions. From "women shouldn't lift heavy weights" to "mood swings are just hormonal," we've heard it all.

Together, we'll debunk these myths. We'll bring in science, expert opinions, and shared experiences from women around the globe. But more than anything, we'll learn to trust our narratives and find our truths.

Embracing the Changes

From the first period to menopause, the female body goes through a plethora of changes. Each phase brings its unique challenges and beauties. Often, society makes us dread these transitions. Remember the hush-hush around getting your first period or the whispered conversations about the dreaded 'M' word (Menopause)?

Instead of dreading them, what if we celebrated these transitions? What if we saw them as badges of honor, as milestones in our incredible journey? This perspective shift is crucial. It's time to embrace the changes, to understand them, and to prepare for them.

Eating, Moving, Thriving: More Than Just Buzzwords

"Eat, Move, Thrive." These three words sum up the essence of this book. But they're more than just catchy phrases. They represent a holistic approach to women's health that we often overlook.

Eat: Think about it. Food isn't just fuel. It's tradition, it's celebration, it's love, it's medicine. Our relationship with food can tell us so much about our relationship with ourselves. Through the chapters, we'll look at how to eat in a way that honors our unique physiology, needs, and yes, our cravings too!

Move: Movement, for us women, is transformative. Whether it's the grace of yoga, the exhilaration of a run, the joy of a dance, or simply a leisurely stroll in the park – the way we move can be a reflection of how we feel. We'll dive into how movement, tailored to our unique needs and life stages, can be a source of strength, healing, and vitality.

Thrive: Now, here's a word that encapsulates our ultimate goal. Thriving isn't just about being disease-free. It's about waking up with zest, having that sparkle in our eyes, feeling connected, joyful, and purposeful. It's about holistic well-being.

A Roadmap Tailored to You

As we embark on this journey together, remember that every woman's experience is unique. While there are common threads that bind our stories, your path is your own. This book aims to be a guide, a companion, but the choices, interpretations, and decisions are yours to make.

You might have moments of profound realization, times when you laugh out loud, or instances where you ponder deeply. Embrace them all. This is your journey of self-discovery, of celebrating the marvel that is you.

And as we turn the pages, imagine us sharing this journey, as friends, as sisters, as fellow explorers. We'll celebrate the victories, navigate the challenges, and savor the wonders of womanhood.

So, my dear reader, are you ready? Let's dive in, learn, and transform. Let's eat, move, and above all, thrive!

With that said, it's crucial to understand that this journey isn't about achieving an "ideal" state of health. Perfection is not the goal. The goal is understanding, compassion, and well-being. It's about celebrating the moments when we feel on top of the world and understanding and caring for ourselves when we don't.

In the chapters to come, we'll unpack each aspect in detail. We'll share stories, facts, laughs, and perhaps a few tears. But through it all, we'll be on this journey together – learning, growing, and celebrating the incredible world of women's health.

With that, dear reader, our journey in "Eat, Move, Thrive: The Female Blueprint" truly begins. From understanding the intricate balance of our hormones to finding joy in movement, from nourishing our bodies with love and care to understanding the deeper layers of our psyche – we're in this together. So, hold tight, the adventure has just begun!

Let's go on this adventure with open hearts and open minds. Here's to celebrating and understanding the marvel that is the female form! Cheers to us!

2 THE PHYSIOLOGY OF FEMINITY: UNDERSTANDING THE FEMALE BODY

Understanding the female body's physiology is fundamental to promoting women's health and well-being. The female body is remarkable in its complexity, and there are several key aspects that deserve attention.

First and foremost, the female reproductive system is a defining feature of femininity. It involves a delicate balance of hormones that regulate the menstrual cycle, which is unique to women. These hormones, such as estrogen and progesterone, play a central role in a woman's health, impacting not only reproduction but also bone density, mood, and overall vitality.

Pregnancy is a transformative experience in a woman's life, and it's crucial to recognize the physiological changes that occur during this time. The body undergoes adaptations to support the growing fetus, from changes in hormone levels to an increase in blood volume and circulation. Adequate prenatal care is essential to ensure the health of both the mother and the developing child.

Menopause is another significant physiological milestone in a woman's life. As women age, hormonal shifts occur, leading to the end of reproductive cycles. These changes can bring about various symptoms like hot flashes and mood swings. Understanding the options for managing these symptoms, including hormone replacement therapy and lifestyle adjustments, is essential.

Breast health is unique to women as well. Regular breast self-examinations and mammograms are vital for early detection of breast cancer, which is a top health concern for women.

Women also tend to have a higher percentage of body fat than men, which can affect metabolism and energy levels. Proper nutrition and exercise tailored to individual needs are essential for maintaining a healthy body composition.

Moreover, women's bodies can respond differently to stress, and hormonal fluctuations can play a role in mood and emotional well-being. Strategies for stress management and emotional health are important considerations in women's overall wellness.

Alright, ladies, grab a comfy seat, maybe a cup of tea or coffee, because we're about to dive deep into the wondrous world that is the female body. If our bodies were novels, this chapter would be all about understanding the core narrative, the plot twists, and the central characters. Ready? Let's go!

Once Upon a Time: The Beginning

Okay, let's take a quick trip down memory lane. Remember those awkward biology classes in middle school? The diagrams, the blush-worthy discussions, and those overly clinical words? Yep, those. Well, think of this as a redo, but this time, we'll chat like friends discussing the latest binge-worthy Netflix series.

The Star of the Show: The Female Reproductive System

Let's begin with the star of our show: the female reproductive system. It's been both celebrated and stigmatized, but here, we're all about celebrating its magnificence.

- **Ovaries:** Think of them as the managers of the entire show. They produce eggs and release hormones like estrogen and progesterone. Oh, and fun fact: by the time we're born, our ovaries already contain all the eggs we'll ever have!

- **Fallopian Tubes:** These are the pathways that guide an egg from an ovary to the uterus. Imagine them as serene little walkways, guiding the future.

- **Uterus:** Ah, the mighty uterus. Every month, it preps a cozy lining for a potential baby. If there's no baby, it discards the lining (hello, periods!). And if there is a baby? Well, it becomes home sweet home for the next nine months.

- **Cervix:** It's like the gatekeeper between the uterus and the vagina. When you hear about Pap smears? They're checking the cervix for any unwelcome changes.

- **Vagina:** The birth canal, the passage, the part of us that's been both mythologized and misunderstood.

It's elastic, it's self-cleaning (whoa, right?), and plays a key role in our sexual health.

Rollercoaster Rides: The Menstrual Cycle

Oh boy, where to begin? The menstrual cycle is like that rollercoaster ride – some days we're soaring high, and other days we're diving deep. It's not just about that 'time of the month.' It's a sophisticated, month-long dance of hormones and processes.

- **Menstrual Phase (Day 1-5):** This is when we bleed. Our body sheds the uterine lining since there's no baby to house. It's also a kind of 'reset' for the next cycle.

- **Follicular Phase (Day 1-13):** Happening simultaneously with menstruation, our body prepares to release another egg. Ovaries are bustling, and estrogen is on the rise.

- **Ovulation Phase (Day 14):** It's go-time! One of the ovaries releases a mature egg, which gracefully sashays down the fallopian tube. It's hoping to meet a sperm, and if it does, conception happens.

- **Luteal Phase (Day 15-28):** Post ovulation, the body preps for a potential pregnancy. The hormone progesterone dominates this phase. If the egg isn't fertilized, estrogen and progesterone levels drop, leading us back to the menstrual phase.

Hormones: The Behind-The-Scenes Crew

Hormones! These are like the backstage crew in a theater production, ensuring everything runs smoothly. From how we feel to the health of our reproductive systems, these little chemical messengers play a HUGE role.

- **Estrogen:** Our very own 'girl power' hormone. It helps develop female physical features, manages our menstrual cycle, and keeps our bones strong.

- **Progesterone:** The sidekick to estrogen, it prepares the body for pregnancy and regulates the menstrual cycle.

- **Testosterone:** Surprise! It's not just a 'male' hormone. In smaller amounts, it plays a role in our bone strength, libido, and mood.

Busting Myths and Embracing Truths

Alright, time for a little myth-busting session.

- **Myth 1:** PMS is just about mood swings. *Reality:* It encompasses a range of symptoms from bloating to headaches, and yes, mood changes. Every woman's PMS experience can be different.

- **Myth 2:** A regular menstrual cycle is strictly 28 days. *Reality:* It varies. For some, it's 21 days, and for others, it can be 35. What's regular is what's consistent for you.

- **Myth 3:** Menopause marks the end of femininity. *Reality:* Absolutely not! It's a new chapter, yes, but it can also be a time of empowerment and renewed energy.

Nourishing and Loving Our Bodies

Our bodies are not just biological systems; they're temples, homes, and sources of immense power.

Understanding our physiology is just the beginning. Nourishing our bodies with love, care, and the right nutrients is crucial. Think of it as watering a plant; with the right care, it thrives and blossoms.

Wrap-Up: Celebrating the Marvel

Ladies, we've journeyed through the marvel that is the female body. From our intricate reproductive systems to the hormonal ballet that happens within us, it's all nothing short of magical.

Remember, the more we understand, the more empowered we become. As we move through this book, we'll delve deeper into how to nourish, nurture, and love our bodies. But for now, let's take a moment to marvel at the magic within us. Here's to celebrating the physiology of femininity!

If you are interested in reading scientific explanation of the chapter, here you go:

The Physiology of Feminity: Understanding the Female Body

Hey there, lovely ladies! Alright, let's dive right into this fascinating journey of understanding the intricate and awe-inspiring world of the female body. Our physiology is an ensemble of art and science, and understanding it can be truly empowering. So, shall we begin?

Once Upon a Time: The Cellular Magic

Each of us began as a single cell, a fusion of our mother's egg and our father's sperm. This zygote, as it's called, carries 46 chromosomes—23 pairs, where one of each pair comes from each parent. The XX chromosomal pairing is what determines the female sex, and it sets the stage for everything that follows in our development.

The Star of the Show: The Female Reproductive System

The female reproductive system isn't just about reproduction; it plays a central role in hormone production, which has wide-ranging effects on our overall health.

- **Ovaries:** These almond-shaped organs are nestled in the pelvic region. Not only do they house our ova (eggs), but they're also our body's primary source of estrogen and progesterone, essential hormones that regulate numerous physiological processes.

- **Fallopian Tubes:** Lined with cilia (tiny hair-like structures), they help usher the egg from the ovaries to the uterus. The fertilization of an egg by a sperm typically occurs in the fallopian tubes.

- **Uterus:** This muscular organ has an impressive ability to expand during pregnancy. Its lining, the endometrium, thickens and sheds during the menstrual cycle. The rich vascularization here provides the needed nutrients to a fertilized egg.

- **Cervix:** Acting as the lower part of the uterus, it produces cervical mucus that changes in consistency during the menstrual cycle to either prevent or facilitate sperm movement.

- **Vagina:** Its muscular walls are lined with mucous membranes that keep it protected and moist. The acidic pH (thanks to beneficial bacteria) helps prevent infections.

The Intricate Ballet: The Menstrual Cycle

The menstrual cycle isn't just a monthly event; it's a carefully coordinated ballet of hormones and physiological processes.

- **Menstrual Phase (Day 1-5):** Shedding of the uterine lining marks this phase. Prostaglandins, a group of lipids, trigger the uterus to contract, helping expel the lining.

- **Follicular Phase (Day 1-13):** The pituitary gland releases Follicle Stimulating Hormone (FSH), prompting the ovaries to produce around five to 20 follicles. Each follicle contains an immature egg.

- **Ovulation Phase (Day 14):** A surge in Luteinizing Hormone (LH) and a smaller increase in FSH leads to the release of a mature egg from the dominant follicle.

- **Luteal Phase (Day 15-28):** The ruptured follicle transforms into a structure called the corpus luteum, which releases progesterone. This hormone prepares the endometrium for a potential implantation.

Hormones: The Symphony Conductors

- **Estrogen:** Beyond reproductive health, it protects against heart disease, supports bone density, and even plays a role in mood regulation. Variations in estrogen levels can impact neurotransmitters like serotonin.

- **Progesterone:** This hormone prepares and maintains the endometrium for a fertilized egg to implant. It also plays a role in breast development and can influence mood and libido.

- **Testosterone:** While it's often termed a "male hormone", females produce it in smaller amounts in the ovaries and adrenal glands. It contributes to libido, muscle strength, and the maintenance of bone density.

Busting Myths and Embracing Science

- **Myth 1:** Only one egg matures each menstrual cycle. *Reality:* While typically only one egg is released, multiple follicles can begin the maturation process, with one becoming dominant.

- **Myth 2:** Ovaries take turns releasing an egg each month. *Reality:* It's random! Either ovary can release the egg in any given month.

- **Myth 3:** Menopause means an end to female hormone production. *Reality:* Even post-menopause, the ovaries continue producing testosterone and small amounts of estrogen.

Nourishing and Respecting Our Bodies

Understanding our intricate physiology underscores the importance of holistic health—be it nutritional, physical, or emotional. As we delve deeper into this book, we'll explore how to best support and cherish our bodies.

In Closing: A Tribute to the Female Physiology

From the cellular choreography that starts in the womb to the hormonal symphonies of our monthly cycles, the female body is a marvel. As we journey through life, understanding and embracing our physiology can empower us to live healthier, more informed lives.

3 NUTRITION 101: THE BASICS EVERY WOMAN SHOULD KNOW

Hello, fabulous women of the world!

Let's delve into the basics of nutrition that every woman should be aware of.

Nutrition is the cornerstone of health and wellness for women. It's essential to understand the fundamental principles to make informed choices about what you eat.

First and foremost, a balanced diet is key. This means consuming a variety of foods from different food groups. Fruits, vegetables, lean proteins, whole grains, and healthy fats should all be part of your daily intake. Each of these provides essential nutrients that your body needs.

Caloric intake is another crucial aspect. The number of calories you need depends on various factors, including age, activity level, and metabolism. It's important not to consume more calories than your body requires to maintain a healthy weight.

Protein is essential for women. It plays a vital role in maintaining muscle mass, supporting the immune system, and repairing tissues. Sources of lean protein include poultry, fish, beans, and tofu.

Calcium is crucial for bone health. Women are at higher risk of osteoporosis, so it's important to get enough calcium through dairy products, leafy greens, or fortified foods.

Iron is vital for women, especially during menstruation. Good sources of iron include red meat, poultry, fish, beans, and fortified cereals.

Folate is essential for women of childbearing age. It helps prevent neural tube defects in babies. You can find folate in leafy greens, citrus fruits, and fortified cereals.

Fiber is important for digestive health and can help manage weight. Foods like whole grains, fruits, and vegetables are excellent sources of dietary fiber.

Hydration is often overlooked but critical. Women should aim to drink plenty of water throughout the day to stay properly hydrated.

Moreover, it's essential to be mindful of portion sizes. Even healthy foods can contribute to weight gain if consumed in excessive amounts.

Lastly, listening to your body is key. Pay attention to hunger and fullness cues, and try to eat mindfully rather than in a rush.

Let's talk food. We all love a decadent chocolate cake or crispy fries once in a while, don't we? But let's face it, nutrition can often be confusing. Carbs? Proteins? Superfoods? What does it all mean? Fear not, by the end of this chapter, we'll be food-wise and ready to make empowering choices. Are you ready to dig in (pun intended)?

Let's go!

The Foundation: Macronutrients

We often hear terms like carbs, fats, and proteins. But what are they, really? These are what we call macronutrients. They're the pillars that support our bodily functions.

- **Carbohydrates:** These are our primary energy source. Remember how you feel all pumped up after a hearty pasta meal? That's the carbs at work!

  - *Types*: Simple carbs (sugars) provide quick energy. Think candies. Complex carbs (like whole grains) release energy slowly, keeping us full and energetic.

  - *Daily Dose*: The Dietary Guidelines for Americans recommend that 45-65% of our daily caloric intake come from carbohydrates. But focus on the good ones – whole grains, veggies, and fruits.

- **Proteins:** Think of them as the building blocks. They help repair tissues, produce enzymes, and are vital for overall growth.

  - *Sources*: Meat, fish, eggs, dairy, legumes, and some grains and veggies.

  - *Daily Dose*: Women should aim for 46-56 grams daily. If you're active or pregnant, you might need more.

- **Fats:** Often villainized, but so essential! Fats insulate our organs, support cell growth, and help in the absorption of certain vitamins.

    - *Types*: Unsaturated (olive oil, nuts), saturated (red meat, butter), and trans fats (some processed foods). Aim for more unsaturated fats and be wary of trans fats.

    - *Daily Dose*: Around 20-35% of your daily calories. For a 2,000-calorie diet, that's about 44-77 grams of fat.

Micronutrients: Vitamins and Minerals Galore

While macronutrients give us energy, micronutrients are about finesse. They ensure the smooth functioning of various bodily processes.

- **Iron:** Essential for the formation of red blood cells.

    - *Why It's Special for Us*: Menstruation can cause iron loss. Thus, getting enough iron is crucial.

    - *Sources*: Red meat, beans, spinach, quinoa, and fortified cereals.

- **Calcium:** A key player for strong bones and teeth.

    - *Why It's Special for Us*: Especially important during puberty and post-menopause to prevent osteoporosis.

    - *Sources*: Dairy products, leafy greens, almonds, tofu, and fortified foods.

- **Folate:** Crucial for cell division and especially important during pregnancy.

    - *Sources*: Leafy greens, citrus fruits, beans, and fortified cereals.

The Fabulous Fibers

Ah, the unsung heroes of the nutrition world. Fibers are a kind of carbohydrate that our bodies don't digest. Yet, they play pivotal roles.

- *Why We Love Them*: They help with digestion, can lower cholesterol levels, and keep us full, aiding in weight management.

- *Sources*: Whole grains, fruits, vegetables, and legumes.

- *Daily Dose*: Aim for 21-25 grams a day.

Water, Water Everywhere!

Our bodies are about 60% water. From aiding digestion to regulating temperature, water does it all.

- *Daily Dose*: About 8 glasses or 2 liters. If you're active or live in a warm climate, you might need more.

What's the Deal with Superfoods?

"Eat chia seeds!", "Have you tried quinoa?", "Blueberries are the secret to life!" We've all heard it. But what's the actual deal with superfoods?

- They're foods dense in nutrients and antioxidants. They're awesome, but remember, no single food can offer all the health benefits we need. So, while we incorporate them, let's not forget the basics.

Deciphering Dietary Guidelines

Every few years, dietary guidelines get a revamp. New research, trends, and understanding shape them. They're a good baseline, but remember, we're all unique. Listen to your body and adjust accordingly.

Supplements: Do We Need Them?

With aisles and aisles of supplements in stores, it's a legit question. Here's the scoop:

- **Multivitamins:** They can be a good backup. But aim to get most nutrients from food.

- **Calcium and Vitamin D:** Especially as we age, these become vital.

- **Iron:** If you're pregnant or have heavy periods, consider this.

Note: Always consult with a healthcare provider before starting any supplements.

Eating for Life Stages

From periods to pregnancies to menopause, our bodies go through so much. Each stage has unique nutritional needs:

- **Teenage Years**: Growth spurts require more of everything – calories, proteins, calcium, and iron.

- **Pregnancy and Breastfeeding**: Needs for iron, folate, and calcium go up.

- **Menopause**: The metabolic rate might slow down. Focus on proteins, calcium, and vitamin D.

Dietary Choices: Vegetarian? Vegan? Pescatarian?

Whatever path you choose, balance is key. Ensure you're not missing out on essential nutrients.

In a Nutshell (Almonds, Preferably!):

Nutrition is not just about numbers or trendy diets. It's about nourishing our bodies and souls. With every bite we take, we're making a choice. Let's make choices that honor our uniqueness and support our journey through the different stages of womanhood.

Ladies, here's to eating well, living well, and thriving!

25

Note: Nutrition is a vast field, and while we covered many basics, always seek personalized advice from nutrition professionals. Your health deserves it!

4 EATING FOR YOUR CYCLE: HOW THE MENSTRUAL CYCLE INFLUENCES NUTRITIONAL NEEDS

Hey there, incredible women of the world!

Understanding how the menstrual cycle affects nutritional needs is a critical aspect of women's health. The menstrual cycle is divided into several phases, each with its unique hormonal changes, and these changes can indeed influence what your body needs.

During the menstrual phase, which is when you have your period, it's common to experience lower energy levels and possible iron loss through blood. Therefore, it's a good idea to focus on foods rich in iron, such as lean meats, beans, and leafy greens, to help combat fatigue and replenish iron stores.

As you move into the follicular phase, which comes after your period, hormone levels start to rise. This is a good time to emphasize a balanced diet with a variety of nutrients. Incorporating plenty of fruits, vegetables, and whole grains can provide essential vitamins and minerals needed for overall health.

The ovulatory phase is when you're most fertile. Hormones like estrogen peak during this time, and your metabolism may increase slightly. It's important to stay hydrated and maintain balanced meals. Including foods rich in antioxidants can also be beneficial for overall well-being.

The luteal phase, which occurs after ovulation and before your next period, is often associated with changes in mood and energy levels. It's common to experience cravings during this phase. Opting for healthy snacks like nuts, yogurt, and dark chocolate can help satisfy cravings without overindulging in less nutritious options.

Calcium intake is essential for women throughout their menstrual cycle, but it's particularly important during the luteal phase when some women may experience PMS symptoms. Dairy products, fortified plant-based milk, and leafy greens can provide calcium to support bone health and potentially ease PMS symptoms.

Listening to your body is crucial. If you find yourself craving certain foods during specific phases of your menstrual cycle, it's okay to indulge occasionally. However, maintaining a balanced diet throughout the month is key to meeting your overall nutritional needs.

Let's talk about something we're all too familiar with but don't often chat about in the context of nutrition – our menstrual cycles. From those teen years to menopause, this monthly guest (for many of us) comes with mood swings, energy shifts, and more. But did you know your menstrual cycle also influences your nutritional needs? Buckle up, we're about to dive deep!

A Quick Refresher on the Menstrual Cycle

Before we go on, let's remember how this magical cycle works:

- **Menstrual Phase (Days 1-5)**: This is when the uterine lining sheds (hello, period).

- **Follicular Phase (Days 1-13)**: The body prepares to release an egg. It's all about the buildup!

- **Ovulation (Day 14)**: An egg is released from the ovary, saying, "Hello world, I'm here!"

- **Luteal Phase (Days 15-28)**: This is the post-egg release phase, leading up to menstruation.

Okay, back to food!

Menstrual Phase: Comfort Food Time?

Ah, those days of cramps, bloating, and perhaps some moodiness. Your body is shedding its lining, and you might feel a tad drained.

- **What's Happening Nutritionally?**: You're losing iron, thanks to the blood loss. Your magnesium levels might be on the dip too.

- **What to Eat**: Think iron-rich foods like spinach, lentils, and red meat. And for magnesium, reach for those almonds, whole grains, and dark chocolate (yes, you read that right!).

Follicular Phase: Energize Me!

This is when things ramp up. Your body is prepping to release that egg, and estrogen levels rise.

- **What's Happening Nutritionally?**: You're probably feeling energetic. Your body is primed for muscle growth and repair.

- **What to Eat**: Lean proteins like chicken, fish, and tofu. Pair it with complex carbs like quinoa and oats to fuel your day. And hey, don't shy away from healthy fats like avocados and olive oil.

Ovulation: Hello, Radiance!

During ovulation, you might feel on top of the world! Radiant skin, peak energy, and perhaps a heightened libido.

- **What's Happening Nutritionally?**: With the surge in luteinizing hormone and follicle-stimulating hormone, your body might crave more zinc.

- **What to Eat**: Indulge in foods rich in zinc such as pumpkin seeds, cashews, and chickpeas. Also, as our bodies are more sensitive to insulin during this phase, try to balance your carb intake with protein.

Luteal Phase: Ride the Rollercoaster

Welcome to the emotional rollercoaster. As progesterone rises, you might experience PMS symptoms like mood swings and cravings.

- **What's Happening Nutritionally?**: Your metabolism is in overdrive! This means you might feel hungrier than usual.

- **What to Eat**: First, B-vitamins are your friend! They can boost mood and energy. So, load up on eggs, fish, and leafy greens. For those carb cravings, choose fiber-rich foods like sweet potatoes and berries. And if you're feeling bloated, foods rich in potassium, like bananas and tomatoes, can help.

Common PMS Symptoms and How to Combat Them with Nutrition

We've all been there, right? Here's a handy guide:

- **Bloating**: Aim for foods rich in potassium and magnesium. Think bananas, oranges, and nuts. And remember, drink water! Counterintuitive, but it helps with bloating.

- **Mood Swings**: Omega-3 fatty acids can be a mood enhancer. So, enjoy some fatty fish like salmon or snack on some walnuts.

- **Fatigue**: Remember iron and B-vitamins. They can provide that much-needed energy lift.

Foods to Potentially Avoid During Certain Phases

- **Menstrual Phase**: Maybe cut back on caffeine. I know, tough. But it can exacerbate breast tenderness and bloating.

- **Luteal Phase**: You might want to minimize salty foods to counteract bloating. And while sugar might be tempting, it can lead to mood crashes.

The Power of Hydration

Throughout your cycle, water is your best buddy. It aids digestion, reduces bloating, and can even help with cramps. So keep that water bottle close!

Why the Right Nutrition Matters

Beyond alleviating PMS symptoms, understanding how to eat for your cycle can:

- Boost energy levels.
- Improve skin health.
- Balance mood and hormones.
- Aid in muscle repair and growth.

Supplements to Consider

While food is queen, sometimes, we might need an extra boost:

- **Iron**: Especially if you have heavy periods.
- **Magnesium**: Can help with cramps and mood swings.
- **Omega-3s**: For mood and inflammation.
- **Vitamin B6**: Can be beneficial for mood regulation.

Always chat with a healthcare provider before diving into supplements.

Final Bites (of Wisdom)

Ladies, our bodies are dynamic. Just as the moon waxes and wanes, our cycles have their rhythms. By tuning into these rhythms and eating to support them, we empower ourselves. We give our bodies what they need when they need it. And in return, we feel better, more balanced, and in sync with our unique female essence.

So, the next time you reach for a snack or plan a meal, think about where you are in your cycle. Honor that phase with nutrition that supports and nourishes. Here's to celebrating every phase of our cycle with the food we eat!

Note: While we've covered a lot here, remember every woman is unique. Always listen to your body, and if needed, seek personalized advice from nutrition professionals. Your health deserves it!

5. STRENGTH IN MOVEMENT: THE POWER AND PURPOSE OF EXERCISE FOR WOMEN

Hey, beautiful women out there!

Exercise holds immense power and purpose for women's health, and it goes far beyond aesthetics. Engaging in regular physical activity is a fundamental aspect of a healthy lifestyle that provides numerous benefits specific to women.

First and foremost, exercise helps build and maintain muscle mass, which is crucial for women as they age. It contributes to overall strength and can significantly improve bone density, reducing the risk of osteoporosis, a condition more prevalent in women.

Physical activity is also instrumental in managing body weight. Women may face unique challenges in this regard, such as hormonal fluctuations, especially during pregnancy and menopause. Regular exercise helps manage weight by increasing metabolism and burning calories.

Moreover, exercise plays a pivotal role in cardiovascular health. Heart disease is a leading cause of death for women, and regular aerobic exercises like brisk walking, jogging, or swimming can help lower the risk of heart disease. It also helps regulate blood pressure and cholesterol levels.

Mood and mental well-being are closely linked to physical activity. Exercise releases endorphins, the body's natural mood lifters, and can help alleviate symptoms of depression and anxiety. It's a powerful stress management tool that many women find invaluable in their daily lives.

For women of childbearing age, exercise can improve fertility and support a healthy pregnancy. Staying active during pregnancy can ease discomfort, improve circulation, and help with postpartum recovery.

Additionally, pelvic floor exercises are essential for women's health. These exercises can help prevent issues like incontinence and support the reproductive organs. Women can incorporate pelvic floor exercises into their routine to maintain pelvic health.

As women go through various life stages, from menstruation to menopause, exercise can help manage the associated symptoms. It can alleviate menstrual cramps, improve sleep quality, and mitigate some menopausal symptoms like hot flashes.

Lastly, exercise fosters a sense of empowerment and confidence. It's not just about physical strength but also mental resilience. Women often find that the discipline and achievement in their fitness journey carry over into other aspects of their lives.

Grab a comfortable seat (or stand if you're feeling the energy!) because we're about to talk about a topic I'm super passionate about: the wonder of women's bodies in motion. It's time we discuss how exercise isn't just about looking a certain way but feeling a powerful connection with our own bodies. So, let's lace up our metaphorical sneakers and get moving!

1. Why Women's Exercise is Special

Wait, what makes our exercise regimen so unique?

Here's the thing: women's bodies, with our hormonal fluctuations, bone structures, and metabolic rates, respond to exercise differently than men's. It's not about who's stronger or better; it's about understanding the nuances of our own physiology to get the most out of every workout.

2. The Hormonal Dance and Exercise

Hormones. We have a love-hate relationship with them, right? But when it comes to exercise, they play a huge role.

- **Estrogen**: Not just for reproduction! It helps in muscle repair and can even influence how we store fat. Knowing this, we can time high-intensity workouts for when our estrogen levels peak for faster muscle recovery.

- **Progesterone**: This can make us feel a bit sluggish, so during its peak times (hello, luteal phase!), you might switch to low-impact exercises.

Tip: Track your cycle and adjust your workouts. Your body will thank you!

3. Strength Training: Not Just for the Boys

Some women fear weight lifting thinking it might make them too 'bulky'. Let's bust this myth now. Women typically have lower testosterone levels, making it hard to bulk up. Instead, lifting weights:

- Improves bone density (super important for post-menopausal women).

- Boosts metabolism.

- Shapes and tones our muscles beautifully.

4. Cardio: Heart Health and Beyond

Cardio isn't just for weight loss. For us, it:

- Boosts lung function.

- Improves heart health (essential as heart diseases can be a concern for older women).

- Releases those feel-good endorphins (who doesn't love the runner's high?).

5. Flexibility and Balance: Embrace the Grace

Yoga, Pilates, and Tai Chi aren't just trendy exercises. They:

- Enhance flexibility (great for joint health).

- Improve balance (which is crucial as we age).

- Connect the mind and body, promoting mental wellness.

6. Pelvic Power: The Core of Being a Woman

Our pelvic floor is the unsung hero of our bodies. It supports reproductive organs and aids in bladder control. Exercises like Kegels strengthen this area, reducing the risk of prolapse and improving sexual health.

7. The Mental Wellness Aspect

Exercise isn't just about the body. The mental benefits are phenomenal:

- **Stress Reduction**: Physical activity increases the production of endorphins, our natural stress-busters.

- **Confidence Boost**: Every time you achieve a new fitness milestone, your confidence gets a lovely boost.

- **Combatting Depression and Anxiety**: Regular exercise can be as effective as medication for some people in reducing symptoms of depression and anxiety.

8. The Social Butterfly Effect

Joining a Zumba class or a hiking group is not just good for our bodies but also our social lives. Making connections, laughing over shared experiences, and having a support system are integral for holistic health.

9. Pregnancy and Exercise

For those expecting or planning to, exercise is still on the cards! It:

- Helps with easier labor.

- Reduces pregnancy-related complications.

- Aids in quicker postpartum recovery.

Remember: Always consult with your OB/GYN before starting any exercise regimen during pregnancy.

10. Menopause and Beyond: Keep Moving!

As we hit menopause, exercise becomes even more critical:

- Bone health: To counteract the risks of osteoporosis.

- Weight management: As metabolism slows down, movement helps in managing weight.

- Mental health: To combat potential mood swings or feelings of depression.

Making Exercise a Habit: Tips for Success

Okay, now that we know the why let's talk about the how:

- **Start Slow**: You don't have to run a marathon tomorrow. Start where you are.

- **Find Your Tribe**: Join classes, find workout buddies, and surround yourself with motivation.

- **Listen to Your Body**: Some days you'll feel the burn; other days, you might need rest. That's okay.

- **Set Goals, Not Just Aesthetically**: Don't just focus on weight loss. Maybe aim for lifting heavier, running longer, or mastering that tricky yoga pose.

Closing Thoughts

Ladies, our bodies are our temples. They tell stories, bear burdens, and create life. And just like any temple, they deserve care, respect, and celebration. Through movement, we honor our bodies, ensuring they serve us robustly and healthily.

Remember, exercise is not about punishment or fitting into societal standards. It's about celebrating what your body can do and pushing it to find new limits. Here's to strength, resilience, and the beautiful dance of femininity in motion! Keep moving, keep shining!.

6 HORMONAL HARMONY: FOODS, EXERCISES, AND LIFESTYLE CHOICES FOR BALANCE

Hey there, wonderful ladies!

let's have a conversational discussion about how foods, exercises, and lifestyle choices can contribute to hormonal harmony for women.

Maintaining hormonal balance is a vital aspect of women's health, influencing everything from mood to metabolism. So, let's dive into how we can support hormonal harmony in everyday life.

Our diet plays a significant role in hormonal balance. It's about nourishing our bodies with the right nutrients. For instance, including fiber-rich foods like whole grains and vegetables helps stabilize blood sugar levels, which is crucial for hormonal health. Healthy fats, found in foods like fatty fish and nuts, are great for supporting hormone production and reducing inflammation. Plus, getting enough protein from lean sources like chicken, beans, and tofu helps regulate hormones.

On the flip side, it's a good idea to limit sugar and processed foods. These can cause insulin spikes, throwing hormones off balance. So, opting for whole, unprocessed foods is a smart choice.

Exercise is a fantastic way to promote hormonal harmony. Aerobic exercises like running or swimming help regulate insulin levels and boost mood. Strength training, meanwhile, supports muscle health, which is essential for hormonal balance. And don't forget about practices like yoga, which can reduce stress, something that can have a significant impact on hormones.

Our lifestyle plays a big role too. Stress, for instance, can wreak havoc on hormones. That's where stress management techniques like meditation or deep breathing can be incredibly helpful. And, of course, getting enough quality sleep is essential. Sleep is when our bodies do a lot of hormone regulating.

It's also a good idea to watch your alcohol and caffeine intake. Overindulging in these can disrupt hormone balance, so moderation is key. Maintaining a healthy weight is important as well, as excess body fat, particularly around the abdomen, can lead to hormonal imbalances.

Lastly, it's essential to be in tune with your own body. Recognize your hormonal patterns and any irregularities. Regular gynecological check-ups are crucial for detecting and addressing any issues like PCOS or thyroid imbalances.

In essence, achieving hormonal harmony is about adopting a holistic approach to your health. It's about making mindful choices in your diet, finding an exercise routine that suits you, managing stress, and listening to your body's signals. When we take care of these aspects, we support hormonal balance and overall well-being.

As we embark on this enlightening journey through the winding world of hormones, let's make a pact. Let's promise to be patient with ourselves, to be kind to our bodies, and to celebrate the little victories along the way. Because trust me, understanding and balancing hormones isn't a sprint; it's a marathon. And with every step we take, we're getting closer to achieving that harmonious balance. Ready? Let's dive in!

1. Hormones 101: A Quick Refresher

Before we dive deep, let's take a quick refresher course on hormones. Picture them as little messengers zipping around inside your body, delivering essential messages that determine everything from your mood, appetite, to how you store fat. They're basically the postal service of the body!

2. Estrogen: The Queen Bee

Why's everyone always talking about estrogen?

Well, because she's kind of a big deal. She plays a massive role in everything from menstruation to bone density. But, as with all things, too much or too little can cause chaos.

Balancing Act:

- **Foods**: Focus on fiber-rich foods like flaxseeds, fruits, and veggies.

- **Exercise**: Cardio helps in lowering high estrogen levels, so time to get that heart rate up!

- **Lifestyle**: Avoiding plastics (like BPA) can help, as they can mimic estrogen in the body.

3. Progesterone: The Unsung Hero

Often in estrogen's shadow, progesterone is equally essential. It regulates the menstrual cycle, prepares the body for pregnancy, and can even affect your mood.

Balancing Act:

- **Foods**: Magnesium-rich foods like nuts, spinach, and bananas.

- **Exercise**: Yoga and Pilates can be beneficial. Relaxation is key!

- **Lifestyle**: Stress can lower progesterone levels. Time to embrace relaxation techniques, be it meditation or a bubble bath.

4. Cortisol: The Stress Messenger

Known as the 'stress hormone', cortisol isn't all bad. It keeps us alert and ready for challenges. But chronic stress means chronic high cortisol, leading to problems like weight gain.

Balancing Act:

- **Foods**: Omega-3 fatty acids found in fish can help reduce cortisol levels.

- **Exercise**: Ever heard of the 'runner's high'? Cardio can help keep cortisol in check.

- **Lifestyle**: Prioritize sleep. Trust me, your cortisol levels will thank you.

5. Insulin: The Energy Regulator

Insulin is all about energy regulation. But imbalances can lead to insulin resistance, often a precursor to diabetes.

Balancing Act:

- **Foods**: Opt for whole grains and minimize sugar. Spikes in blood sugar can mess with insulin.

- **Exercise**: Strength training can increase insulin sensitivity.

- **Lifestyle**: Small, frequent meals throughout the day can help stabilize insulin.

6. Thyroid Hormones: The Metabolic Managers

These powerhouses regulate our metabolism, energy, and body temperature. But if they're out of whack? Hello, fatigue and unexplained weight changes.

Balancing Act:

- **Foods**: Seaweed and other iodine-rich foods support the thyroid. But be mindful, as too much can backfire.

- **Exercise**: Consistency is key. Even brisk walking can make a difference.

- **Lifestyle**: Manage stress and regularly check with your doctor if thyroid issues run in your family.

7. Testosterone: Not Just For Men

Surprise! Women have testosterone too, influencing muscle mass, bone density, and even mood.

Balancing Act:

- **Foods**: Zinc-rich foods like shellfish and beans can help in its production.

- **Exercise**: Weightlifting can give you a testosterone boost.

- **Lifestyle**: Limit alcohol. It can decrease testosterone levels.

8. Connecting Diet and Hormonal Balance

Let's chat about foods that promote hormonal balance, and no, it's not just broccoli:

- **Phytoestrogens**: Found in foods like soy, they can mimic estrogen in the body. Handy for those with low estrogen.

- **Healthy Fats**: Think avocados, olive oil, and nuts.

- **Cruciferous Veggies**: Broccoli, cauliflower, and their gang can help regulate estrogen.

9. Moving to Balance

Exercise is fantastic for hormonal harmony:

- **Mix It Up**: Combine cardio, strength training, and flexibility workouts.

- **Listen to Your Body**: Some days you might want an intense HIIT session, others a calming yoga flow. That's okay.

10. The Lifestyle Factor

Finally, lifestyle tweaks can make a world of difference:

- **Mindfulness and Meditation**: Yes, it's not just a trend. It genuinely helps.

- **Limiting Toxins**: Be it in skincare or cleaning products, be mindful of endocrine disruptors.

Wrap-Up: Finding YOUR Balance

While all these tips are general guidelines, remember, every body is unique. What works wonders for one might not work for another. So, keep experimenting, be patient, and remember: you're not alone on this journey. With every bite, every step, and every deep breath, you're working towards your unique hormonal harmony. Celebrate that journey, embrace the process, and remember to enjoy every moment. Your harmonious self awaits!

(P.S. Always consult with a healthcare provider before making significant changes to your diet or exercise routine!)

Alright, ladies, that's a wrap on this chapter. I hope it shed some light on the intricate dance of our hormones and how we can nourish and nurture them. Until next time, keep glowing, growing, and flowing in your own unique rhythm. Onward and upward!

7 WEIGHT MANAGEMENT AND METABOLISM: MYTHS, REALITIES, AND STRATEGIES

Hey there, superstar!

There are plenty of myths and realities to explore in this topic, along with some strategies that can help.

First off, metabolism – it's a term that gets thrown around a lot, but what exactly is it? Your metabolism is basically the process your body uses to convert what you eat and drink into energy. It's influenced by factors like age, gender, genetics, and muscle mass.

Now, one common myth is that some people just have a fast metabolism and can eat whatever they want without gaining weight. While it's true that genetics play a role, the impact isn't as massive as you might think. Your metabolism can be influenced and improved by lifestyle choices.

Another myth is the idea of "starvation mode." Some believe that eating too little can slow down your metabolism, making it harder to lose weight. In reality, extreme calorie restriction can slow down metabolism temporarily, but it's not a sustainable or healthy way to manage weight.

On the flip side, it's not all about eating less to lose weight. Crash diets and severe calorie restriction can lead to muscle loss, which actually slows down metabolism. So, it's not just about the quantity of calories you eat but also the quality.

What's important is finding a balance that works for you. Focus on a balanced diet that includes a variety of foods, with an emphasis on fruits, vegetables, lean proteins, and whole grains. This helps keep your metabolism running smoothly and provides the nutrients your body needs.

Exercise is another key player in the metabolism game. Muscle burns more calories than fat, so strength training can help boost your metabolism. Plus, physical activity, in general, helps you maintain a healthy weight and supports overall well-being.

Consistency is vital when it comes to weight management. Quick fixes and fad diets might show short-term results, but they're often not sustainable. It's better to make gradual, long-term changes to your eating and exercise habits. That way, you're more likely to maintain a healthy weight over time.

Remember that it's okay to seek support. A registered dietitian or a personal trainer can provide personalized guidance and help you set realistic goals. They can also help you navigate the sea of information and myths surrounding weight management and metabolism.

In essence, weight management and metabolism are complex, but they're not mysterious. It's about finding a balance that works for you, making healthy choices, and being patient with yourself. Quick fixes rarely lead to lasting results, so focus on the long-term journey to a healthier you.

Let's chat about a topic many of us have had a love-hate relationship with: weight management. Toss in metabolism, and you've got a cocktail of confusion, myths, and countless diet fads. Take a deep breath. Let's demystify this together and arm you with knowledge that *actually* matters.

1. What's the Deal with Metabolism?

Simply put, metabolism is your body's energy-burning process. Think of it as an internal furnace, turning the food you eat into the energy you need. Factors like age, muscle mass, and genetics play a role in how fast (or slow) this furnace burns.

2. Myth: Thin People have High Metabolism; Overweight People have Low Metabolism

Let's debunk this right off the bat. Metabolic rate is not solely dependent on body size or weight. In fact, larger bodies often burn more calories even at rest because they need more energy to function.

3. The Basal Metabolic Rate (BMR) Riddle

BMR is the rate at which we burn calories while resting (yeah, even while you're binge-watching your fave show). Factors influencing BMR:

- Age
- Gender
- Muscle mass
- Hormonal factors

4. Myth: Starvation Mode – Eating Less Means Metabolism Slows Down, Right?

It's not that black and white. While drastically reducing calories can decrease metabolic rate, it's usually not to the "starvation" extent most diets warn about. However, consistently consuming very few calories isn't a sustainable or healthy weight management strategy.

5. Muscle Mass: The Unsung Hero of Metabolism

Muscle tissue burns more calories than fat, even when you're at rest. The takeaway? Strength training is your friend, lovely!

6. Breakfast: The Metabolic Jumpstart?

You've heard it: "Breakfast is the most important meal." But is skipping it slowing your metabolism? Not necessarily. Listen to your body. Some folks thrive on breakfast, while others feel better fasting until later. Find what works for you.

7. Myth: "Boost Your Metabolism" Foods

Green tea, chili peppers, coffee – can they really rev up your metabolism? While some foods and drinks *might* give a tiny, temporary boost, they're not magic. Enjoy them, but don't rely on them solely for weight management.

8. Drinking Water for the Win!

Studies suggest that drinking water can temporarily boost metabolism by about 10-30%. Plus, it's great for overall health and can help you feel full.

9. Sleep: The Unsung Metabolic Hero

Poor sleep can mess with the hormones that regulate appetite and lead to weight gain. Treat your sleep like gold, darling.

10. The Reality of Set Point Theory

Your body has a weight range it's comfy at, and it'll resist efforts to change it, be it gaining or losing. It's frustrating, but knowing about it can help you set realistic expectations.

11. Small, Frequent Meals: Yay or Nay?

Some swear by it for metabolism boosting; others shrug. The science? It might help, but it's more about total caloric intake over the day. The key is consistency and quality.

12. Stress: The Silent Metabolic Saboteur

When stressed, your body releases cortisol, which can prompt fat storage, especially around the midsection. Deep breaths, self-care, and maybe some yoga can help.

13. Weight Loss Supplements & Metabolism Boosters

Be cautious. While tempting, many of these have limited evidence backing them and can have side effects.

14. Diet Types & Metabolism

Keto, intermittent fasting, low-carb, vegan – each has its pros and cons. The best diet? One that you can maintain, that nourishes you, and makes you feel vibrant.

15. Listening to Your Body: The Ultimate Strategy

Tuning into your hunger cues, energy levels, and how foods make you feel is priceless. It's more reliable than any diet trend.

16. Celebrate Non-Scale Victories

Your worth isn't tied to a number. Celebrate improved energy, better sleep, clothes fitting differently, and feeling stronger.

17. Seeking Professional Guidance

Sometimes, we need a helping hand. Whether it's a nutritionist, doctor, or therapist, don't hesitate to seek guidance.

Alright, beautiful soul, that's our journey through weight management and metabolism. Remember, amidst all the science and strategies, the most important thing is to love and nurture yourself. Weight is just a number; your well-being is the entire story. Stay radiant and empowered!

8 NAVIGATING MENOPAUSE: DIET, EXERCISE, AND WELL-BEING TIPS

Menopause is a unique phase in a woman's life, and it can come with its fair share of changes. But it's essential to remember that it's a natural transition, and there are ways to make it more manageable.

Hey there, fabulous lady! ✨ Ready to talk about a phase in life that sometimes feels like Mother Nature's curveball? Menopause. A journey, a transition, an *adventure* — call it what you will. Let's navigate this path with grace, understanding, and a good dose of humor. Grab a cup of your favorite tea (or wine; we won't judge), and let's dive in.

1. The M-Word: What Exactly IS Menopause?

Just to level set: menopause isn't a single event or a disease. It's a natural phase where your periods come to an end, and you can no longer conceive naturally. It's your ovaries saying, "We've clocked out." But you're far from done. In fact, many say life begins anew!

2. Symptoms & Changes: What's the 411?

From hot flashes and night sweats to mood swings, sleep disturbances, and *ahem* a drier 'lady garden'. It's not the same for everyone, so let's empower ourselves with knowledge and the right tools.

3. Eating Right: Food as Fuel and Friend

- **Phytoestrogens**: Found in soy products, flax seeds, and whole grains, these can be a gal's best friends, mimicking the effects of estrogen in the body.

- **Calcium & Vitamin D**: As bone density can decrease, it's essential to consume foods rich in calcium and Vitamin D. Think leafy greens, dairy, and fortified foods. Sun, anyone?

- **Omega-3s**: Great for brain health and combatting mood swings. Get these from fatty fish, walnuts, and chia seeds.

- **Stay Hydrated**: Water is key. It helps with dry skin and keeps everything 'flowing' (if you catch my drift).

4. Exercise: Keep That Body Moving and Grooving!

A sedentary lifestyle? Not on our watch.

- **Strength Training**: As we age, muscle mass can decline. Let's reverse that trend.

- **Aerobics**: Great for heart health and those pesky hot flashes.

- **Flexibility**: Yoga and Pilates can help maintain joint health and relieve stress.

- **Balance Exercises**: Crucial as our balance can become a bit wobbly with age.

5. Hot Flash SOS: Tips & Tricks

- Dress in layers. You'll thank yourself.

- Stay cool with a portable fan or cold drink.

- Note triggers: Sometimes spicy foods or caffeine can set off a flash.

6. Sleep: Claiming Back the Night

- **Routine**: Try going to bed and waking up at the same time each day.

- **Cool Environment**: Helps counteract night sweats.

- **Limit Stimulants**: Reduce caffeine and heavy meals close to bedtime.

7. Mental Well-being: Embrace the Change

- **Mindfulness and Meditation**: Ground yourself. Be present.

- **Talk About It**: Share experiences with friends or consider therapy.

- **Hobbies**: Rekindle old passions or discover new ones. It's *your* time.

8. Libido: The Ups and Downs

Menopause might cause a dip in libido, but that doesn't mean the end of intimacy.

- **Communicate**: Talk with your partner.

- **Stay Adventurous**: Explore new ways of being intimate.

- **Lubricants**: They can be game-changers.

9. Hormone Replacement Therapy (HRT): The Lowdown

It's not for everyone, but it can be beneficial. Chat with your doc about potential risks and rewards.

10. Natural Supplements and Alternative Therapies

From Black Cohosh to Acupuncture, there are numerous routes you can explore. Again, a conversation with a health professional is key.

11. Embrace & Celebrate: Menopause as a New Beginning

Yes, it's a transition. But it's also a chance to reinvent, rediscover, and rejoice in the woman you are.

To wrap up our heart-to-heart, remember: Menopause isn't about loss; it's about change. And just like every phase before this, you've got the strength, wisdom, and sass to handle it brilliantly. Cheers to you, vibrant and ever-evolving woman!

9 OSTEOPOROSIS AND BONE HEALTH: BUILDING AND MAINTAINING STRONG BONES

Hello, dear reader!

Our bones form the foundation of our body, supporting us throughout life. Maintaining bone health is essential, and osteoporosis, which weakens bones and makes them prone to fractures, is a significant concern, especially with age.

Nutrition plays a crucial role. Eating a balanced diet is fundamental for bone health. Calcium is a critical element in building and maintaining strong bones, found in dairy products, fortified plant-based milk, and leafy greens. Vitamin D is equally important as it aids calcium absorption. You can get it from sunlight and foods like fatty fish and fortified cereals. Don't overlook protein; it's necessary for overall bone health and can be found in lean meats, beans, and nuts.

Exercise is another key factor. Engaging in weight-bearing exercises like walking, jogging, and dancing is beneficial. These activities stimulate bone formation and preserve bone density. Strength training, using weights or resistance bands, is also effective in building muscle and fortifying bones.

Lifestyle choices can impact bone health. Quitting smoking and moderating alcohol consumption can significantly impact bone health. Smoking can reduce bone density, and excessive alcohol can hinder calcium absorption.

Balancing and maintaining good posture can help prevent falls, a common cause of fractures in older adults. Practices like yoga and tai chi can enhance coordination and balance, reducing the risk of falls.

Regular check-ups are essential. Bone density screenings, especially for postmenopausal women and older adults, can help detect osteoporosis early, making it easier to manage. Discuss screening recommendations with your healthcare provider.

In severe cases of osteoporosis, medication may be necessary. Consult with your healthcare provider to determine if this is appropriate for you.

Are you ready to embark on a deep dive into one of the most critical yet overlooked aspects of women's health? That's right, today we're chatting about the very framework of our bodies - our bones. So, let's dive into osteoporosis and bone health, and let me let you in on a little secret: It's NEVER too early or too late to start caring for your bones!

1. Bone Basics: What's All the Buzz About?

Did you know your bones are living, breathing tissues? Far from the inert skeletal props we see at Halloween, our bones are constantly being broken down and rebuilt.

Think of them as a never-ending construction site - and osteoporosis? That's when the demolition crew gets a tad overzealous.

2. Osteoporosis 101: More than Just 'Brittle Bones'

While osteoporosis is often dubbed the "silent disease" because you can't *feel* your bones getting weaker, it's no ghost story. It's real. But with awareness and proactive steps, we can take the reins on our bone health journey.

3. Risky Business: Who's At Risk?

Age, family history, early menopause - there are many factors that can up our risk. But, knowing is half the battle, right? Time to play detective with our own health.

4. Food for Thought (and Bones!): Nutrition's Role in Bone Health

- **Calcium**: It's the bone-building superstar! Dairy products, leafy greens, and fortified foods are great sources.

- **Vitamin D**: The sidekick calcium needs to work its magic. Our main source? Sunshine! Plus, some foods and supplements.

- **Protein**: Essential for bone strength. Lean meats, beans, lentils, and tofu are all fabulous choices.

- **Micronutrients Galore**: Magnesium, zinc, vitamin K, and vitamin C also join the party. A varied diet's the key.

5. Move It or Lose It: Exercise for Bone Vitality

Not all exercise is created equal when it comes to bones.

- **Weight-bearing exercises**: Think walking, jogging, dancing, and weightlifting. These beauties put pressure on the bones, signaling them to grow stronger.

- **Balance activities**: Tai chi or yoga can help reduce the risk of falls, a major no-no for fragile bones.

6. Medication Station: When Diet and Exercise Aren't Enough

There are various osteoporosis medications on the market. Some help build bone, while others prevent bone loss. It's all about finding what's right for *you*, under a doctor's guidance, of course.

7. Lifestyle Choices: Small Steps, Big Impact

- **Limit Alcohol & Caffeine**: Overconsumption can reduce calcium absorption. Moderation is key.

- **No Smoking**: Cigarettes can decrease bone density. Yet another reason to ditch the habit!

- **Keep it Light**: Maintain a healthy weight. Being too thin can increase your risk.

8. Bone Density Tests: The Crystal Ball of Bone Health

Consider it a sneak-peek into the future of your bone health. It's a simple scan that can offer so much insight.

9. Preventing Falls: Safety First!

Let's be real: falls can be a major party pooper, especially with weakened bones. Non-slip mats, good lighting, handrails... minor tweaks, major benefits!

10. Embracing Bone Health: It's a Lifelong Journey

From our first steps to our golden years, our bones carry us through life's adventures. Let's ensure they have the strength and vitality to keep the journey thrilling.

Closing our chapter (see what I did there?), remember that bone health isn't just about the now, it's about the future. Imagine dancing at your grandchild's wedding, trekking up mountains in your 70s, or just rocking that pair of heels because, why not? That future starts with the bone choices you make today. So here's to sturdy bones and a life lived fully!

10 HEARTFELT HEALTH: CARDIOVASCULAR WELLNESS FOR WOMEN

Hey there, fabulous reader!

Your heart is a remarkable organ, tirelessly pumping blood and oxygen throughout your body. Taking care of your heart is essential for overall well-being, and it's especially important for women as they have unique considerations when it comes to heart health.

Diet plays a significant role in heart health. A balanced diet rich in fruits, vegetables, whole grains, and lean proteins can help keep your heart in good shape. Try to limit saturated and trans fats, as well as sodium (salt). These can contribute to high blood pressure and heart disease. Instead, opt for healthy fats like those found in nuts, seeds, and fatty fish.

Regular physical activity is like a magic potion for your heart. It helps maintain a healthy weight, reduces stress, and lowers the risk of heart disease. Activities like brisk walking, swimming, or dancing are excellent choices. Aim for at least 150 minutes of moderate-intensity exercise per week, as recommended by health experts.

Stress can take a toll on your heart. Finding healthy ways to manage stress, whether it's through meditation, yoga, or spending time with loved ones, can be incredibly beneficial.

Women should be aware of certain risk factors that can affect heart health. These include high blood pressure, high cholesterol, diabetes, and smoking. Regular check-ups with your healthcare provider can help monitor and manage these risks.

Hormonal changes, especially during menopause, can impact heart health. It's a good idea to discuss these changes with your healthcare provider to determine the best approach for your cardiovascular wellness.

Your family's medical history can also provide important insights. If you have a family history of heart disease, inform your healthcare provider, as it may affect your risk factors and require more vigilant monitoring.

Surround yourself with a supportive network of friends and family who encourage your heart-healthy choices. Additionally, staying informed about heart health through reliable sources can empower you to make the best decisions for your well-being.

In essence, "Heartfelt Health" for women is about taking proactive steps to protect your heart. It's a holistic approach that involves making smart dietary choices, staying active, managing stress, and being aware of your unique risk factors. By doing so, you can nurture a healthy heart and enjoy a vibrant life.

Grab your favorite cozy blanket and a cup of herbal tea, because today, we're diving deep into a topic that's literally close to our hearts: cardiovascular health. You see, our heart does so much more than fuel sappy love songs or beat faster when our favorite actor appears on screen. It's the epicenter of our health, and today, we're giving it the love and attention it so rightly deserves.

1. The Heart of the Matter: Understanding Our Tickers

Alright, here's a fun fact to kick things off: a woman's heart beats faster than a man's. Yep! It's smaller but oh-so-mighty. Our heart pumps blood, which carries essential nutrients and oxygen to every nook and cranny of our bodies.

2. Cardiovascular Diseases (CVD): The Unwanted Guests

CVD encompasses a family of heart-hustling diseases like coronary artery disease, heart failure, and arrhythmias. The not-so-fun truth? Women have unique risks and symptoms. But knowledge is power, my friend.

3. Risk Factors: The Usual (and Not-So-Usual) Suspects

Age, family history, and high blood pressure are on the usual suspects list. But did you know pregnancy complications or menopause can also affect heart health? The plot thickens!

4. Diet Do's and Don'ts: Eat Your Heart Out (the Right Way)

- **Fiber up!** Whole grains, fruits, and veggies are the name of the game.

- **Omega-3s for the win**: Think fatty fish, chia seeds, and walnuts.

- **Easy on the salt**: Let's keep that blood pressure in check, shall we?

- **Cheers to moderation**: Red wine may have heart benefits, but moderation is our mantra.

5. Get Moving, Gorgeous: Exercise and Heart Health

Heart health and exercise go hand in hand. Whether you're dancing in your living room or taking brisk morning walks, every bit counts. Plus, endorphins, anyone?

6. Stress and the Heart: More than Just a Feeling

Chronic stress can lead to heart issues. The good news? Meditation, journaling, or even a cat meme can help dial down those stress levels.

7. Women-Specific Factors: Pregnancy, Menopause, and the Pill

Hormones, pregnancy, birth control, menopause – they don't just affect mood swings or hot flashes. They have direct tickets to the heart show, influencing blood pressure, cholesterol, and more.

8. Diagnostic Tests: Listening to Our Hearts

From ECGs to stress tests, these tools help decode the whispers (or sometimes loud protests) of our hearts.

9. Treatment Options: Modern Miracles

Medications, surgeries, lifestyle changes - today's treatment options are vast and tailored, offering rays of hope and longer, healthier lives.

10. The Mind-Heart Connection: Emotions that Stir the Heart

Did you know intense emotions can cause heartbreak syndrome, where the heart temporarily enlarges and doesn't pump well? It's not just in the movies!

11. A Heartfelt Conclusion: Prioritizing Heart Health

Our hearts are the unsung heroes of our bodies. They beat tirelessly, ask for little, and give so much. By nurturing our heart health, we're not just avoiding diseases; we're embracing life, love, and every beautiful moment that comes with it.

There you have it, lovely reader. A tour of our wondrous hearts and how to care for them. Remember, every beat counts, and it's never too early or late to start heart-healthy habits. So here's to long walks, hearty laughs, and a lifetime of heartfelt moments!

11 MENTAL WELLNESS AND MINDFUL EATING: NUTRITION'S ROLE IN COGNITIVE HEALTH

Hey there, fellow life navigator!

Our mental well-being is closely tied to what we eat. It's not just about physical health but also about nourishing our brains. Here are some key aspects to consider:

Diet: A well-balanced diet can have a significant impact on cognitive health. Foods rich in antioxidants, like fruits and vegetables, help protect brain cells from damage. Omega-3 fatty acids found in fatty fish, flaxseeds, and walnuts are crucial for brain function. And don't forget about whole grains; they provide a steady supply of energy for the brain.

Hydration: Staying hydrated is vital for overall health, including cognitive function. Even mild dehydration can affect mood and cognitive abilities. So, be sure to drink enough water throughout the day.

Mindful Eating: Mindful eating is about paying full attention to your eating experience. It involves savoring each bite, eating slowly, and being in tune with your body's hunger and fullness cues. This approach can help prevent overeating and promote a healthier relationship with food.

Protein: Including enough high-quality protein in your diet is essential. Protein provides amino acids that are the building blocks for neurotransmitters, which are chemicals that transmit signals in the brain. Lean sources like poultry, fish, beans, and tofu are good options.

Sugar and Processed Foods: Limiting sugar and highly processed foods is crucial. They can lead to blood sugar spikes and crashes, affecting mood and cognitive function. Opt for natural sweeteners like honey or maple syrup and choose whole, unprocessed foods whenever possible.

Variety: Eating a variety of foods ensures you get a broad spectrum of nutrients that support brain health. Different foods offer different vitamins, minerals, and antioxidants, so mix it up in your diet.

Moderation: It's not about deprivation but about balance. Enjoying treats in moderation is absolutely fine and can contribute to your overall well-being.

Emotional Eating: Be mindful of emotional eating, where you turn to food for comfort or to cope with stress. Seek healthier ways to manage emotions, like talking to a friend, practicing relaxation techniques, or engaging in a favorite hobby.

You know that unmistakable feeling when you walk into a room and suddenly can't remember why? Or when that word you were about to say just slips off the tip of your tongue? We've all been there. Today, we're pulling back the curtains on the wonder that is our brain, and how what we put on our plate impacts what's happening up in our gray matter. So, let's take this delightful journey into the world of mindful eating and mental wellness, shall we?

1. Brain Food 101: What's on the Menu?

The brain, believe it or not, is a pretty greedy organ, gobbling up around 20% of the energy we consume daily. It's like the high-maintenance friend of our bodily organs. Here's a quick rundown of its favorite snacks:

- **Omega-3 fatty acids**: Found in fish, walnuts, and flaxseeds.
- **Antioxidants**: Blueberries, dark chocolate, spinach... yum!
- **Vitamin E**: Think nuts and seeds.

2. Mind-Gut Connection: Trusting Your Gut Feelings

Ever had a 'gut-wrenching' experience? That's your brain and gut, chatting away. A healthy gut, filled with friendly bacteria, can help fend off anxiety, depression, and even stress. Probiotic-rich foods? Yes, please!

3. Hydration Nation: Watering Our Thinking Caps

Here's a riddle: it makes up about 75% of our brain, and we can't live without it? Water! Staying hydrated doesn't just quench thirst; it boosts cognition and mood. So, bottoms up!

4. The Sugar-Coated Truth: The Highs and Lows of Sugar on the Brain

Ah, sugar. It's the sweet siren song in our favorite treats. But too much can lead to mood swings, foggy thinking, and even depression. Balance, as they say, is sweet!

5. Caffeine Chronicles: A Tale of Love and Alertness

For many, the day doesn't start until that first sip of coffee. And while caffeine can sharpen our alertness, it's a love affair best enjoyed in moderation.

6. Mindful Eating: More than Just a Buzzword

Mindful eating is like giving your meals the attention they truly deserve. It's savoring each bite, being present, and truly tasting your food. And the perks? Reduced stress, better digestion, and a happier you.

7. Emotional Eating: The Comfort Food Conundrum

Stressed spelled backward is desserts. Coincidence? Emotional eating is real, but understanding our triggers and finding healthier coping mechanisms can make all the difference.

8. Brain-Boosting Recipes: A Culinary Adventure

From Omega-3 rich salmon to antioxidant-packed berry smoothies, there's a smorgasbord of foods that love our brains as much as our taste buds.

9. Foods on the Watchlist: Not All Heroes Wear Capes

Certain foods might seem harmless but can impact our mental wellness. From processed foods to those with artificial sweeteners, being informed is half the battle.

10. A Toast to Alcohol: The Good, the Bad, and the Bubbly

A glass of wine might seem relaxing, and in moderation, it can be. But it's essential to understand alcohol's broader effects on our mood and cognition.

11. Spice Up Your Life: Herbs and Spices with Brain Benefits

Turmeric, rosemary, sage – they're not just for seasoning. These wonder herbs and spices can give our brains that extra oomph.

12. Wrapping it Up: Food for Thought

Our brain, magnificent as it is, relies heavily on the menu we provide. As we feed our bodies, we nourish our minds. It's a dance of well-being that starts with every bite, every sip, and every mindful moment.

Well, my insightful reader, there you have it—a hearty serving of knowledge about the deep connection between our brains and our bites. Here's to more mindful munching, delightful dining, and, of course, brainy brilliance! Cheers to good food and even better moods!

12 EMPOWERMENT THROUGH ENDURANCE: CARDIO TRAINING FOR EVERY AGE

Hey there, wonderful reader!

Cardiovascular exercise, often known as cardio, is a fantastic way to boost your physical and mental well-being. It strengthens your heart, reducing the risk of heart disease, which is essential for everyone, especially as we age. Engaging in regular cardio workouts can increase your energy levels, boost stamina, and reduce fatigue.

Cardio training is excellent for managing your weight. It burns calories and helps shed excess pounds or maintain a healthy weight. Cardiovascular exercise triggers the release of endorphins, those feel-good hormones, reducing stress, anxiety, and symptoms of depression.

Many people find that regular cardio workouts lead to improved sleep quality, essential for overall well-being. While cardio primarily targets your heart and lungs, it also engages muscles and contributes to overall strength.

Social opportunities arise from cardio activities like group fitness classes or team sports, fostering connections and a sense of community. Regular cardio training has been linked to a longer, healthier life, helping you stay active and independent as you age.

You can tailor your cardio routine to suit your age and fitness level, whether it's brisk walking, cycling, swimming, or dancing. If you're new to exercise or have underlying health concerns, consult a healthcare provider or fitness professional for a safe and effective cardio plan.

So, you're looking to get that heart racing, aren't you? We're not talking about that swoon-worthy scene from your favorite rom-com. Nope, we're diving deep into the realm of cardiovascular (or cardio) training! Whether you're a spry teen, a magnificent middle-ager, or a gracefully aging senior, this chapter is your golden ticket to understanding and embracing the cardio life. Ready to hit the ground running? Let's jog right in!

1. Let's Talk Cardio: What's All the Buzz About?

Cardio, in its essence, is all about getting that heart rate up. Whether you're dancing, jogging, swimming, or even brisk walking, if your heart's in it, you're doing it right! It's our body's way of saying, "Hey, I'm working here!" And the benefits? Oh, where do we even start: improved heart health, boosted mood, calorie burn, and a lot more.

2. Teen Trailblazers: Cardio in Those Energetic Years

Remember those teenage years? Full of zest and seemingly boundless energy. At this age, the world of cardio is like an open playground! From sports to dance classes, it's all about finding what sets your soul on fire and running (or dancing or swimming) with it.

3. The Fabulous '20s and '30s: Finding Your Cardio Groove

Ah, the roaring twenties and the thrilling thirties! It's a whirlwind of life changes. Work, maybe family, and possibly little ones running around. It might feel challenging to squeeze in that cardio, but this is where short, high-intensity workouts can be your BFF. Ever tried HIIT? It might just be your jam!

4. Rocking the '40s: Adapt and Overcome

Our fabulous forties can often bring about changes in stamina and metabolism. But fear not! This is the perfect time to embrace activities like brisk walking, cycling, or even joining a Zumba class. And, let's not forget about the importance of warming up and cooling down. Trust us; your muscles will thank you!

5. Sailing Through the '50s and Beyond: Grace, Grit, and Cardio

Who says the fifties and onward aren't for cardio? Toss that misconception out the window! It's all about listening to your body and adapting. Water aerobics, tai chi, and dancing can be wonderfully gentle yet effective. Remember, age is just a number; it's the spirit that counts!

6. Mixing It Up: The Key to Cardio Commitment

Routine can be comforting, but when it comes to cardio, variety is the spice of life. Changing things up not only keeps boredom at bay but challenges different muscles and boosts overall endurance.

7. No Gym? No Problem! Home Cardio Solutions

No gym membership? That's hardly a hurdle. From staircase workouts to living room dance-offs, there are countless ways to get that heart rate up right in the comfort of your home.

8. Tools of the Trade: Gear Up for Success

The right shoes, breathable clothing, and perhaps a trusty water bottle. The right gear can make a world of difference, ensuring you get the most out of your cardio sessions while staying comfy and safe.

9. Listen to Your Heart (and Body!): Safety and Limitations

Just as with any exercise regimen, it's vital to stay tuned into our body's signals. Know when to push and when to rest. Stay hydrated, and always, always prioritize safety.

10. Wrapping Up: Your Endurance Empowerment Journey

And there we have it! The world of cardio, demystified and laid out just for you. From the energetic teenage years to the golden ages, there's a cardio rhythm for every soul. As you lace up those sneakers or dive into that pool, remember that every heartbeat, every step, every drop of sweat is a testament to your strength and endurance.

Well, lovely reader, it's time to step, jump, or dance into your cardio adventure. Whether you're sprinting through life's marathons or taking a gentle stroll, remember that every movement is a step towards a heart-healthy, empowered you. Let's get that heart racing for all the right reasons!

13 STRENGTH AND FLEXIBILITY: EMBRACING YOGA AND PILATES

Hello, amazing reader!

Both yoga and Pilates offer a multitude of benefits, including enhanced physical strength, flexibility, improved core stability, better posture, reduced stress, and a strong mind-body connection. These practices are accessible to individuals of various ages and fitness levels due to their low-impact nature. Moreover, they come in various styles and can be customized to meet specific goals, whether it's relaxation, strength-building, or rehabilitation. Engaging with qualified instructors is advisable, especially for newcomers or those with health concerns, to ensure a safe and effective practice that can empower individuals to embrace a healthier and more balanced lifestyle.

Guess what? We're diving into the realm of serenity, strength, flexibility, and grace. I can already hear you saying, "Sounds dreamy!" And you're not wrong. Today, we're unraveling the magic behind two of the most empowering practices on the planet: Yoga and Pilates. Are you ready to get your zen on? Grab a mat, and let's flow together.

1. A Little Backstory: Yoga and Pilates Origins

Before we roll out our mats, let's embark on a tiny time-travel adventure. Yoga, with its roots deep in ancient India, is not just about physical postures; it's a spiritual journey. Meanwhile, Pilates had a more modern beginning, crafted in the early 20th century by Joseph Pilates, focusing on core strength and rehabilitation. Both unique, both powerful!

2. Breathing: The Lifeline of Both Practices

Take a deep breath in... now let it out. Breathing, while a natural process, takes center stage in both Yoga and Pilates. In Yoga, it's known as "Pranayama," bringing life force into our bodies. Pilates, too, has specialized breathing techniques that help activate your core. The key takeaway? Breathe, and let magic unfold.

3. Building Core Strength: Pilates to the Rescue!

Do you ever dream of having a strong, stable core? Who doesn't, right? Pilates is your golden ticket! With its focus on controlled movements and core engagement, you'll not only achieve better posture but also that inner strength you've been yearning for.

4. Yoga: The Blend of Flexibility and Mindfulness

While Yoga does wonders for flexibility (hello, supple spine!), its beauty lies in its union of mind, body, and soul. Whether you're in a deep stretch or holding a challenging pose, it's that inward journey and mindfulness that truly transforms.

5. The Many Faces of Yoga: From Hatha to Hot!

The world of Yoga is vast and varied. Hatha, Vinyasa, Yin, Kundalini, and Hot Yoga, to name a few. Each style offers something unique, from gentle stretches to vigorous flows. The best part? There's a style for every soul out there.

6. Pilates Platforms: Mat vs. Reformer

Pilates isn't just about those mat exercises. Have you heard of the reformer? It's a specialized machine that uses springs for resistance, amplifying the core-engaging benefits of Pilates. Both mat and reformer sessions have their perks, so why not give both a whirl?

7. Combining the Best of Both Worlds

What if you're in love with both Yoga and Pilates? Well, dear reader, meet Yogilates, a blend that brings you the flexibility of Yoga and the core strengthening of Pilates. Talk about a win-win!

8. Setting Up Your Sacred Space

Whether it's a corner in your living room or a dedicated studio space, creating an environment that resonates with tranquility and positivity can elevate your practice to new heights. Think soft lighting, aromatic candles, and maybe some calming tunes.

9. Embracing the Journey, Not the Destination

It's not about nailing that complex pose or perfecting a Pilates move on day one. Embrace the journey, celebrate the small victories, and remember: it's the progress and the learnings along the way that truly count.

10. In Conclusion: Your Path to Strength and Serenity

And there we are, standing at the crossroads of strength, flexibility, and inner peace. Whether you lean towards

Yoga, Pilates, or a blend of both, remember that each breath, stretch, and core engagement is a step closer to a stronger, more flexible, and empowered you.

So, lovely reader, are you ready to embark on this transformative journey? Dive deep, explore, and let the blend of strength and flexibility mold you into the best version of yourself. After all, as they say in Yoga, "The light in me honors the light in you." Namaste and happy practicing!

14 THE GUT-BRAIN CONNECTION: NUTRITION FOR A HEALTHY GUT MICROBIOME

Hey there, savvy reader!

The gut-brain connection is a complex and powerful relationship between your digestive system and your brain. It turns out that what you eat can have a significant impact not only on your physical health but also on your mental well-being.

Your gut is home to trillions of microorganisms, collectively known as the gut microbiome. These tiny residents play a crucial role in digesting food, absorbing nutrients, and even influencing your mood and cognitive function.

The food you consume directly affects the composition of your gut microbiome. A diet rich in fiber, fruits, vegetables, and whole grains promotes a diverse and healthy microbiome. These foods provide the nourishment that beneficial bacteria need to thrive.

Surprisingly, the state of your gut can influence your mental health. A balanced and thriving microbiome can help regulate mood and reduce the risk of conditions like anxiety and depression.

Nutrition also plays a role in controlling inflammation in the gut. Chronic inflammation can negatively impact both physical and mental health. Anti-inflammatory foods like fatty fish, nuts, and colorful fruits and vegetables can help keep inflammation in check.

Probiotics are live bacteria found in foods like yogurt, kefir, and sauerkraut. They can introduce beneficial bacteria into your gut. Prebiotics, found in foods like garlic, onions, and bananas, provide nourishment for these friendly bacteria.

Achieving a healthy gut microbiome is about balance. It's not just about adding probiotics but also about providing them with the right fuel through a varied and fiber-rich diet.

It's worth noting that the ideal diet for gut health can vary from person to person. Some foods may be better tolerated than others, and genetics can play a role in how your gut responds to different nutrients.

In essence, the gut-brain connection underscores the importance of nourishing your body with a balanced and varied diet rich in whole, unprocessed foods. By taking care of your gut microbiome through proper nutrition, you're not only promoting physical health but also supporting mental well-being. It's a powerful reminder of the profound link between what's on your plate and how you feel in both body and mind.

Remember the last time you had 'butterflies in your stomach' when you were nervous or that gut feeling when something wasn't quite right? What if I told you those weren't just expressions but an actual reflection of one of the most exciting areas of scientific discovery: the gut-brain connection?

Welcome to the intricate world of your gut microbiome, where trillions of tiny critters have a massive impact on your overall well-being, especially your brain! Let's deep-dive into this fascinating connection.

1. Setting the Stage: Meet Your Gut and Brain

Imagine two close pals chatting over a coffee. That's your gut and brain, constantly communicating and influencing one another. Your gut, lovingly termed your 'second brain,' has its own nervous system called the enteric nervous system. This system communicates directly with your brain, and the messages go both ways!

2. Microbiome 101: The Mini Metropolis Inside You

Your gut houses trillions of microorganisms – bacteria, fungi, viruses. Think of it as a bustling city with different neighborhoods, each housing its unique residents. The key? Maintaining a harmonious balance for this city to flourish!

3. Mood Food: How Gut Health Influences Your Emotions

Ever felt that post-lunch slump or the happiness from indulging in chocolate? There's science behind that! Certain bacteria in the gut produce neurotransmitters, chemicals that our brain cells use to communicate. Some of these, like serotonin (the happiness hormone), predominantly originate from our gut.

4. Nutrition's Role: Nourishing the Good Bacteria

Not all heroes wear capes; some are found on your dinner plate! Foods rich in fiber, like whole grains, fruits, and veggies, are prebiotics that fuel our good bacteria. Fermented foods, on the other hand, bring in probiotics, introducing beneficial strains directly to our gut.

5. Let's Chat Fermentation: Yogurt, Sauerkraut, and More!

Kombucha, kimchi, miso – the world of fermented foods is vast and delicious. Rich in probiotics, these foods are a boon for gut health, boosting the diversity and abundance of our friendly bacteria.

6. Friendly Fats: Omega-3 and its Role in Gut-Brain Communication

Did you know that Omega-3 fatty acids found in fish, flaxseeds, and walnuts can help support a healthy gut lining, ensuring that gut signals to the brain are crystal clear? So, that salmon dinner isn't just tasty but also brain-friendly!

7. The Dark Side: Sugar, Junk Food, and the Gut-Brain Chaos

Ah, the sweet allure of sugar and processed food. However, indulging too often can cause an imbalance in our gut city, favoring harmful bacteria and leading to foggy thinking and mood swings.

8. Gut Health and Cognitive Function: Clear Gut, Clear Mind

The gut-brain link isn't just about mood. There's growing evidence that a healthy gut microbiome plays a role in maintaining cognitive functions, memory, and even possibly delaying the onset of neurodegenerative diseases. Mind-blowing, right?

9. Inflammation: The Bridge Between Diet, Gut, and Brain

Unhealthy food choices can lead to gut inflammation, which in turn might affect the brain. Chronic inflammation has been linked to mood disorders and even depression. The lesson? Eat right, keep inflammation at bay, and your brain stays happy.

10. A Symphony of Signals: The Vagus Nerve

Connecting your gut and brain is the vagus nerve, the body's information superhighway. By keeping our gut healthy, we ensure that the signals traveling via the vagus nerve to our brain are positive, harmonious tunes rather than distress calls.

In Conclusion: Nurturing Your Inner Ecosystem

Alright, intrepid explorer of the gut-brain universe, here's our takeaway: A happy gut equals a happy brain. By choosing foods that nourish our microbiome, we not only boost our digestion and immunity but also our mental well-being.

So, the next time you're contemplating that plate of veggies or that fizzy probiotic drink, remember you're not just eating for one, but trillions! Let's raise a toast (of kombucha, perhaps?) to a harmonious gut-brain relationship and a happier, healthier you. Cheers!

15. STRESS, SLEEP, AND SERENITY: ACHIEVING BALANCE IN A BUSY WORLD

Hey there, lovely reader!

How to find balance amid stress, prioritize sleep, and cultivate serenity for overall health and well-being.

Stress is a natural part of life, but chronic stress can take a toll on your health. Finding effective ways to manage stress is crucial. This might include techniques like mindfulness meditation, deep breathing exercises, yoga, or even spending time in nature. The key is to find what works best for you and make it a regular practice.

Quality sleep is often underestimated, but it's a cornerstone of good health. Aim for 7-9 hours of sleep per night, as recommended for adults. A consistent sleep schedule and creating a relaxing bedtime routine can help you achieve better sleep. Avoiding screens before bed and creating a comfortable sleep environment are also important.

Your diet plays a significant role in your stress levels and sleep quality. Avoid excessive caffeine and sugar, especially in the hours leading up to bedtime. Instead, opt for foods that support relaxation, such as herbal teas, whole grains, and foods rich in magnesium, like nuts and leafy greens.

Regular exercise is a powerful stress reducer and can promote better sleep. Aim for at least 150 minutes of moderate-intensity exercise per week. This could be as simple as brisk walking, cycling, or dancing.

Learning to manage your time effectively can reduce stress and create space for relaxation. Prioritize your tasks, set realistic goals, and don't be afraid to delegate or say no when necessary.

Spending time with friends and loved ones can provide emotional support and a sense of belonging, which can reduce stress. Make time for meaningful social connections in your life.

Engaging in practices that bring you joy and serenity is essential. This could be reading, playing a musical instrument, gardening, or any hobby you love. These activities can help you unwind and recharge.

If stress and sleep issues persist, don't hesitate to seek help from a healthcare provider or therapist. They can offer guidance, support, and, if necessary, treatment options.

In a world that often seems to demand more of our time and energy, finding balance and prioritizing self-care is vital. Remember that achieving balance is a personal journey, and what works for one person might not work for another. It's about discovering the strategies and practices that resonate with you and integrating them into your daily life to promote overall health and serenity.

You've probably heard the term 'balance' thrown around a lot lately, haven't you? In our fast-paced world, juggling work, family, and personal pursuits often feels like a circus act. Amidst this whirlwind, we're trying to snatch moments of peace, ensure we're getting quality shut-eye, and somehow manage the stress beast that perpetually looms.

Guess what? It's time to pull back the curtains and uncover the secrets of achieving that elusive balance. So, grab your favorite cozy blanket, maybe a cup of calming tea, and let's dive in!

1. The Modern-Day Dilemma: Why Are We So Stressed?

Let's face it: Our ancestors never had to worry about unread emails or social media notifications. Evolutionarily speaking, we're wired for different stressors. But the daily grind, societal pressures, and the always-online culture? It's a lot for our brains to process.

2. Stress: Not All Bad, But Definitely Overstaying its Welcome

Stress is natural. It's our body's response to challenges, releasing hormones like adrenaline and cortisol to tackle the situation. While it's meant to be a temporary state, in today's world, stress has become a constant companion, leading to various health issues.

3. Sleep: The Unsung Hero of Well-being

Ever pulled an all-nighter and felt utterly disoriented the next day? Sleep isn't just "rest"; it's when our body repairs, recharges, and regroups. The world might glorify 'burning the midnight oil', but let's get real: sleep is non-negotiable.

4. Sleep Deprivation: More than Just Yawns and Coffee Binges

A lack of sleep affects mood, cognition, and even our metabolism. And guess what? It's also a major stress amplifier! It's a cycle: stress can affect sleep, and lack of sleep can increase stress. Yikes!

5. Embracing Calm: Techniques to Lower Stress

From deep breathing exercises to grounding techniques, there's an entire toolkit at your disposal. And trust me, it doesn't require meditating atop a mountain. It's about finding what works for you – be it journaling, a calming app, or simple mindfulness practices.

6. Nurturing Nighttime: Tips for Quality Sleep

Good sleep hygiene goes beyond comfy pillows. It's about setting a routine, optimizing your environment (darkness is your friend), and maybe even dabbling in calming pre-sleep rituals. Lavender, anyone?

7. Diet's Role in Stress and Sleep

You are what you eat, and it's truer than you think! Caffeine, sugar, and alcohol can disrupt sleep, while foods rich in magnesium, tryptophan, and certain teas can promote relaxation. Remember, food isn't just fuel; it's medicine.

8. The Serenity Connection: Physical Activity and Mental Peace

Ever heard of the 'runner's high'? Physical activity releases endorphins, our body's natural stress-relievers.

Whether it's a dance class, a brisk walk, or yoga, movement can be a pathway to peace.

9. The Digital Detox: Unplugging for Well-being

Our devices, as useful as they are, often bombard us with stress-inducing stimuli. Designating tech-free zones or times can profoundly impact sleep quality and overall serenity.

10. Building a Resilient Mindset

Life will always have its ups and downs, but building resilience helps us navigate challenges with grace. Strategies like gratitude journaling, cognitive reframing, and seeking social connections can fortify our mental well-being.

In Conclusion: Crafting Your Personal Blueprint for Balance

Here's the thing: There isn't a one-size-fits-all solution. Your path to stress management, restful sleep, and serene moments will be uniquely yours. And that's the beauty of it!

It's a journey of self-discovery, of tuning in and listening to what your body and mind truly need. As we wrap up, remember that balance isn't about perfection. It's about creating a life where stress, sleep, and serenity coexist harmoniously, helping you thrive in this oh-so-busy world.

To calm nights, sunny mornings, and a life lived with purpose – we've got this!.

16 FUNCTIONAL FITNESS: TAILORING EXERCISE TO DAILY LIFE

Hey there, wonderful reader!

Let's chat about functional fitness, a concept that's all about getting your body ready for real-life activities and movements. It's not just about aesthetics; it's about being strong and capable for your everyday life.

Think about those everyday movements like squatting to pick something up, carrying groceries, or reaching for things on a high shelf. Functional fitness focuses on exercises that mimic these actions, making you more efficient and less prone to injuries in your daily routine.

A strong core is a cornerstone of functional fitness. It's not just about looking good; it's about having a stable core that supports your spine and helps prevent injuries.

Functional fitness workouts involve multiple muscle groups and joints, which enhances your balance, coordination, and overall body awareness.

Flexibility and mobility are equally important. It's about having the freedom to move comfortably, bend, twist, and reach without discomfort.

The beauty of functional fitness is that it can prevent injuries by strengthening the muscles and joints you use in your everyday tasks.

No matter your fitness level, you can benefit from functional fitness. It's adaptable and can be tailored to your specific needs and goals.

Plus, it's enjoyable because it incorporates a variety of movements, making workouts engaging and dynamic.

The ultimate goal of functional fitness is to make your daily life easier and more enjoyable. Whether it's playing with your kids, doing household chores, or simply moving without pain, functional fitness can significantly improve your quality of life.

If you're new to it or have any health concerns, consider consulting with a fitness professional. They can help you create a personalized program that fits your needs and goals.

In a nutshell, functional fitness is about preparing your body for life's adventures, making you strong, agile, and capable in your daily activities. It's a practical and enjoyable way to lead a healthier and more active life, no matter your age or fitness level.

Okay, hands up if this sounds familiar: You've been going to the gym, pumping iron, nailing that treadmill, and doing those fancy exercises you saw online. You feel stronger, and your muscles look defined. But then, one day, you bend down to pick up a heavy bag, or you're trying to reach a top shelf, and - *ouch!* - you pull something.

Why? Because while isolated exercises are great for muscle definition and some specific goals, they might not always translate into real-world strength and mobility. Enter: Functional Fitness.

1. Decoding 'Functional Fitness'

At its core, functional fitness is about training your body to handle real-life situations. Think of it as your daily-life bootcamp – exercises that mimic and prepare you for everyday activities, ensuring that you're strong, balanced, and agile where it truly counts.

2. The Daily Grind: Movements We Take for Granted

From getting out of bed, lifting objects, pushing doors, to climbing stairs - our day is filled with repetitive movements. Functional fitness ensures these actions are pain-free and efficient.

3. The Foundations of Functional Fitness

- **Stability**: Before you can jump or lift, you need a stable base. This often comes from your core – not just those abs, but the deep muscles that wrap around your spine.

- **Mobility**: It's all about range! Can your joints move freely? This is especially crucial for areas like our shoulders and hips.

- **Strength**: But not just any strength – functional strength. This is about compound movements and full-body exercises.

4. The Functional Favorites: Exercises that Pack a Punch

- **Squats**: Think about how often you sit and stand. This movement is a daily essential.

- **Lunges**: A lunge is essentially a step, intensified. Great for balance and leg strength.

- **Push-ups**: Beyond just chest strength, a good push-up engages your core, arms, and even legs.

- **Pull-ups**: Mimicking the action of pulling something down or lifting oneself up.

- **Deadlifts**: Lifting something from the ground? That's a deadlift in real-life.

5. The Perks: Why Go Functional?

Apart from being incredibly practical, functional fitness can lead to fewer injuries, better posture, improved balance, and enhanced overall strength. It's the kind of fitness that genuinely aids your daily life.

6. Merging Functional with Traditional

You don't need to abandon your current regimen. It's about integrating functional movements, ensuring that your fitness routine has a healthy mix catering to both aesthetics and practicality.

7. The Gear: Tools to Elevate Your Functional Training

- **Kettlebells**: Oh, the versatile joy of kettlebells! Swings, lifts, and goblet squats - there's a lot to explore.

- **Resistance Bands**: These stretchy wonders can add resistance to almost any movement, enhancing strength and mobility.

- **Stability Balls**: Perfect for core workouts and improving balance.

8. Personalizing Your Functional Regime

Your daily life, chores, and challenges are unique. Maybe you have kids you're constantly lifting, or perhaps your job requires more bending and stooping. Your functional fitness routine should reflect your life and its demands.

9. Setting Up Your Functional Fitness Space

While many functional exercises require minimal equipment, having a dedicated space can boost motivation. Even a small corner with a mat, resistance bands, and a kettlebell can do wonders!

10. The Functional Finale: Evolve and Assess

The beauty of functional fitness is its adaptability. As your strength and mobility improve, your exercises should evolve. Regularly assess how you feel during daily activities and adjust accordingly.

In Conclusion: Life's a Playground, Play Functionally

Functional fitness is like giving yourself the tools to navigate life's physical challenges with ease and confidence. So the next time you're lifting a suitcase, playing with your kids, or doing garden work, know that your body is prepared and primed.

Ready to make daily life your gym? Let's get functionally fit together and celebrate every squat, lift, and stretch that makes life a little easier and a lot more fun!

17 SUPERFOODS FOR THE SUPER WOMAN: BOOSTING HEALTH WITH POWER-PACKED FOODS

Hey there, amazing soul!

You know how in comic books, heroes have their special source of power, like Spiderman with his radioactive spider or Wonder Woman with her divine origin? Well, what if I told you that you, too, have a set of superpowers waiting for you, hidden in the foods you eat?

That's right! Today, we're diving into the fantastic world of superfoods. And trust me; by the end of this chapter, you'll want to integrate them into your diet faster than Superman can fly!

1. Super... what now? Defining 'Superfoods'.

Superfoods don't wear capes, but they're real heroes. These are nutritionally dense foods that deliver more health bang for your caloric buck. They're loaded with vitamins, minerals, antioxidants, and more!

2. Blueberries: The Antioxidant All-Star

Small, blue, and mighty! Blueberries are jam-packed (pun intended!) with antioxidants that help counteract free radicals in our bodies. These tiny fruits can help with aging, boost cognitive function, and support heart health.

3. Quinoa: The Ancient Grain

Oh, quinoa, how we love thee! This grain is an excellent protein source, containing all nine essential amino acids. Plus, it's gluten-free, making it a go-to for many!

4. Avocado: The Fat We All Love

Gone are the days when fats were foes. Avocados are rich in healthy monounsaturated fats. They're also loaded with fiber, potassium, and vitamin K. And hey, who can resist a good guacamole?

5. Kale: The Leafy Green Giant

This might be the Hulk of leafy greens. It boasts vitamins A, K, and C, alongside fiber, calcium, and other minerals. Smoothies, salads, chips - kale fits everywhere.

6. Almonds: Small but Mighty Nuts

Heart-healthy fats, fiber, and protein - almonds have it all. They can help manage weight, provide sustained energy, and even support brain health.

7. Turmeric: Nature's Golden Healer

Curcumin, an active ingredient in turmeric, has potent anti-inflammatory properties. It's no wonder turmeric teas and lattes are becoming a popular health elixir!

8. Chia Seeds: The Tiny Powerhouses

Rich in fiber, omega-3 fatty acids, and protein, chia seeds are a great addition to yogurts, smoothies, and puddings. They also help in digestion and can support heart health.

9. Dark Chocolate: Yes, It's Good for You!

Oh, sweet joy! Dark chocolate, especially with 70% cocoa or more, is loaded with antioxidants. It can help reduce heart disease risk and, let's admit, elevate our mood instantly!

10. Salmon: The Omega-3 Star

Salmon isn't just delicious; it's a fantastic omega-3 fatty acid source. These fatty acids can help reduce inflammation, lower blood pressure, and benefit heart health.

11. Integrating Superfoods: Daily Dose of Awesomeness

Now, the trick is not just knowing about these foods but incorporating them into your daily meals. Whether it's a blueberry smoothie at breakfast, a quinoa salad for lunch, or a salmon dinner, the options are endless.

12. Superfoods are Super, but Diversity is the Key

Remember, while these foods are fantastic, variety is crucial. Make sure you're consuming a diverse range of nutrients by mixing up your food choices regularly.

13. Quick Superfood Recipes for the Busy Woman

No time? No problem! I'll share some quick and tasty recipes to ensure you get your superfood fix without a fuss.

Superfood Recipes for the Busy Woman

1. Blueberry-Almond Smoothie Bowl

Ingredients:

- 1 cup blueberries (frozen or fresh)
- 1/2 banana
- 1 tbsp chia seeds
- 1/4 cup almonds
- 1 cup almond milk
- A handful of granola (for topping)

Instructions:

- In a blender, combine blueberries, banana, chia seeds, almonds, and almond milk until smooth.
- Pour into a bowl and top with granola. Enjoy!

2. Quick Quinoa Salad

Ingredients:

- 1 cup cooked quinoa (cooled)
- 1/2 cup cherry tomatoes (halved)
- 1/4 cup chopped kale
- 1/4 cup feta cheese
- 2 tbsp olive oil
- 1 tbsp lemon juice
- Salt and pepper to taste

Instructions:

- Mix quinoa, cherry tomatoes, chopped kale, and feta cheese in a bowl.

- Drizzle with olive oil, lemon juice, salt, and pepper. Toss to combine and serve!

3. Avocado Toast with a Twist

Ingredients:

- 1 ripe avocado

- 2 slices of whole grain bread

- 1/2 tsp turmeric

- Pinch of chili flakes

- Salt to taste

- 1 tbsp chia seeds (for sprinkling)

Instructions:

- Mash the ripe avocado in a bowl. Mix in turmeric, chili flakes, and salt.

- Toast the bread slices until golden.

- Spread the mashed avocado mixture on the toast. Sprinkle with chia seeds. Relish!

4. Chocolate Chia Seed Pudding

Ingredients:

- 1/4 cup chia seeds

- 1 cup almond milk

- 2 tbsp cocoa powder

- 1-2 tbsp honey or maple syrup

- A pinch of salt
- Fresh berries for topping

Instructions:

- In a bowl, whisk together chia seeds, almond milk, cocoa powder, honey or maple syrup, and salt until well combined.
- Refrigerate for at least 4 hours, or overnight.
- Before serving, give it a good stir, top with fresh berries, and indulge!

5. Salmon Kale Wraps

Ingredients:

- 2 grilled salmon fillets (pre-cooked)
- 4 kale leaves (large)
- 1/2 avocado (sliced)
- 1/4 cup plain yogurt
- 1 tsp lemon zest
- Salt and pepper to taste

Instructions:

- Lay out the kale leaves flat on a plate.
- Place half a salmon fillet on each kale leaf.
- Add avocado slices on top of the salmon.
- In a small bowl, mix yogurt, lemon zest, salt, and pepper. Drizzle this over the salmon and avocado.
- Roll the kale leaves carefully to make a wrap. Secure with a toothpick if needed.

6. Turmeric Golden Milk

Ingredients:

- 2 cups of milk (can use almond, coconut, or regular milk)
- 1 tsp turmeric powder
- A pinch of black pepper
- 1/2 tsp cardamom powder
- 1 tbsp honey or jaggery

Instructions:

- In a pot, heat the milk but avoid bringing it to a boil.
- Add turmeric, black pepper, and cardamom.
- Simmer for 5 minutes, stirring occasionally.
- Remove from heat, sweeten with honey or jaggery. Sip warm!

7. Spinach and Paneer Salad (Palak Paneer Salad)

Ingredients:

- 1 cup paneer (cottage cheese), cubed
- 2 cups spinach leaves, washed and chopped
- 1/2 cup cherry tomatoes, halved
- 1/4 cup roasted walnuts, crushed
- 1/2 tsp cumin powder

- 1 tbsp lemon juice
- Salt to taste

Instructions:

- Toss paneer cubes in a heated non-stick pan until they're golden on all sides.
- In a large bowl, combine the spinach, cherry tomatoes, and roasted paneer.
- Drizzle with lemon juice, sprinkle cumin powder, and salt. Mix well.
- Top with crushed roasted walnuts. Serve fresh!

8. Ragi (Finger Millet) Porridge

Ingredients:

- 1/2 cup ragi flour
- 2 cups water
- 1/2 cup grated jaggery
- A pinch of cardamom powder
- Chopped nuts for garnish

Instructions:

- Mix ragi flour in a half cup of water to make a smooth paste.
- Bring the rest of the water to boil and slowly add the ragi paste, stirring continuously.
- Once it starts thickening, add jaggery and cardamom. Mix until well combined.
- Serve hot, garnished with chopped nuts.

9. Amla (Indian Gooseberry) Juice

Ingredients:

- 4-5 fresh amlas
- 2 cups of water
- 1 tbsp honey
- A pinch of salt or chat masala

Instructions:

- Remove the seeds from the amlas and chop them into smaller pieces.
- Blend the amla pieces with water until smooth.
- Strain the juice, add honey and a pinch of salt or chat masala. Stir well and drink fresh!

10. Chia and Mango Lassi

Ingredients:

- 1 cup yogurt
- 1/2 cup ripe mango pulp
- 2 tbsp chia seeds
- 1 tbsp honey (optional)
- A pinch of cardamom powder

Instructions:

- Mix chia seeds with 1/4 cup of water and let it sit for 10-15 minutes.
- Blend yogurt, mango pulp, soaked chia seeds, honey, and cardamom until smooth.
- Serve chilled with a sprinkle of chia seeds on top.

11. Quinoa Pulao with Vegetables

Ingredients:

- 1 cup quinoa, rinsed
- 2 cups water or vegetable broth
- 1 onion, finely chopped
- 1 carrot, diced
- 1 bell pepper, chopped
- 1/2 cup peas
- 2 tbsp oil or ghee
- 1 tsp cumin seeds
- 1/2 tsp turmeric powder
- 1/2 tsp red chili powder (adjust to taste)
- 1/2 tsp garam masala
- Salt to taste
- Fresh coriander leaves for garnish

Instructions:

- Heat oil or ghee in a pan and add cumin seeds. Once they splutter, add the onions and sauté until translucent.
- Add the diced vegetables and stir-fry for a few minutes.
- Add the quinoa, turmeric, red chili powder, and salt. Mix well.
- Pour in the water or vegetable broth. Bring the mixture to a boil.
- Reduce the heat to low, cover, and simmer until quinoa is cooked and all the water is absorbed.

- Fluff with a fork, sprinkle garam masala and garnish with fresh coriander leaves. Serve hot with yogurt or raita.

12. Beetroot & Spinach Paratha

Ingredients:

- 2 cups whole wheat flour
- 1 beetroot, grated
- 1 cup spinach, finely chopped
- 1 green chili, finely chopped (optional)
- 1/2 tsp cumin powder
- Salt to taste
- Water, as needed for the dough
- Ghee or oil, for frying

Instructions:

- In a large mixing bowl, combine the flour, grated beetroot, chopped spinach, green chili, cumin powder, and salt.
- Knead the mixture into a soft dough by gradually adding water.
- Divide the dough into equal-sized balls.
- Roll each ball into a round paratha with the help of a little flour.
- Heat a tawa or skillet and cook each paratha with ghee or oil until golden brown on both sides.
- Serve hot with pickle, yogurt, or a side of fresh salad.

13. Coconut & Chia Seed Pudding

Ingredients:

- 3 tbsp chia seeds
- 1 cup coconut milk
- 1 tbsp jaggery or honey
- 1/2 tsp cardamom powder
- Fresh fruit slices (like mango, banana, or berries) for topping
- Toasted coconut shreds for garnish

Instructions:

- In a bowl, mix chia seeds and coconut milk. Let it sit for about 30 minutes, or until the mixture becomes gelatinous.
- Add jaggery or honey and cardamom powder. Mix well.
- Pour the mixture into serving bowls or glasses.
- Top with fresh fruit slices and sprinkle toasted coconut shreds.
- Chill in the refrigerator for at least 2 hours before serving.

14. Bajra (Pearl Millet) Khichdi

Ingredients:

- 1 cup bajra, soaked overnight
- 1/2 cup moong dal (yellow split lentil)
- 3 cups water
- 1 tsp cumin seeds

- 1/4 tsp asafoetida (hing)

- 1/2 tsp turmeric powder

- 1/2 tsp red chili powder

- Salt to taste

- 2 tbsp ghee

- Fresh coriander leaves and grated ginger for garnish

Instructions:

- Heat ghee in a pressure cooker or deep pot. Add cumin seeds and asafoetida.

- Once the cumin seeds crackle, add the soaked bajra and moong dal.

- Add turmeric, red chili powder, and salt.

- Pour water and mix everything well.

- If using a pressure cooker, cook for 4-5 whistles. If using a pot, cover and cook on low heat until both bajra and dal are soft.

- Garnish with fresh coriander leaves and grated ginger. Serve hot with a dollop of ghee on top.

In Conclusion: Unleashing Your Inner Wonder Woman

With these superfoods in your arsenal, you're not just feeding your body; you're nurturing your very essence. They are nature's way of saying, "Hey, I've got your back!"

Ready to feel invincible? Start your superfood journey today, and watch as you transform, feeling more energetic, radiant, and empowered. Superfoods for the Super Woman – that's the mantra!

18 THE SKIN YOU'RE IN: NUTRITION AND EXERCISE FOR HEALTHY SKIN

Hey there, beautiful Ladies!

Your skin is like a mirror reflecting your inner health. Here's how what you eat and how you move can make a difference:

Drinking enough water keeps your skin hydrated and looking plump. It's like giving your skin a refreshing drink from the inside.

Foods rich in antioxidants, like colorful fruits and veggies, protect your skin from damage and keep it looking youthful. Omega-3 fatty acids found in foods like salmon and flaxseeds maintain your skin's moisture and fight inflammation. Nutrients like vitamin C, E, and zinc found in various foods support your skin's health and appearance. Collagen, the protein that keeps your skin firm, needs a good supply of protein in your diet. So, lean meats, fish, tofu, and legumes are your friends.

Exercise gets your blood flowing, delivering essential nutrients to your skin cells. That's how you get that healthy glow. Lower stress levels from regular exercise can mean fewer breakouts and skin issues. Stress isn't a friend to your skin.

Sweating during workouts helps clear out toxins, which can be good news for your skin's clarity. Strength training exercises can tone your muscles, which can help your skin look firmer, especially as you age. Enjoy your outdoor workouts, but remember sunscreen. Protecting your skin from the sun's rays is essential.

Don't forget to drink water during and after exercise. It's crucial for skin health. A balanced diet, regular exercise, and a good skincare routine all contribute to glowing skin. Avoiding excessive sugar and processed foods also helps keep your skin looking its best.

You know, they often say our skin is a mirror, reflecting our overall health. I couldn't agree more! How often have you heard someone say, "You're glowing!" when you're feeling good on the inside? That's because our skin, the body's largest organ, often showcases our health from the inside out. But here's the exciting part: What if I told you that the foods you eat and the way you move can influence that glow? Let's dive in and chat about the intricate connection between what we consume, how we exercise, and the health of our skin.

1. The Nutritional Glow-Up

Remember those days when mom used to say, "Eat your greens; they're good for you"? Well, turns out, she was onto something.

Antioxidants – Nature's Skin Protectors:
Foods high in antioxidants, like blueberries, spinach, and even dark chocolate (yay!), help protect our skin from the damaging effects of free radicals. Think of antioxidants as your skin's personal bodyguards, fighting off those unruly free radicals.

Hydration is Key:
Your skin craves hydration. Besides drinking ample water, indulge in foods with high water content. Think watermelon, cucumber, oranges, and strawberries. Not only do they quench your thirst but also keep your skin plump and youthful.

Omega-3 Fatty Acids:
Hello, glowing skin! Foods like walnuts, chia seeds, and fatty fish are loaded with omega-3s. They help maintain cell membranes, allowing for optimal nutrient absorption and waste removal.

Collagen Boosters:
Vitamin C-rich foods like bell peppers, guavas, and citrus fruits aid in collagen production, ensuring skin stays firm and wrinkle-free. Collagen peptides and bone broth are also gaining popularity as skin-nourishing supplements.

2. Exercise – More than Just Breaking a Sweat

Exercise isn't just for those rock-hard abs; it's also for that soft, glowing cheek!

Increased Blood Flow:
Working up a sweat increases blood flow, ensuring essential nutrients get to our skin. So, the next time you're jogging, know that you're also giving your skin a treat.

Stress Reduction:
Ever noticed breakouts when you're stressed? Exercise,

especially yoga and meditation, can reduce cortisol levels (that pesky stress hormone), leading to clearer skin.

Post-exercise Glow:
That post-workout glow isn't a myth. The dilation of blood vessels during a workout gives the skin a rosy, healthy appearance. But remember to cleanse post-exercise to remove any sweat and bacteria.

3. Foods to Embrace and Foods to Avoid

Say YES to:

- **Bright Veggies:** Carrots, bell peppers, and tomatoes are not just colorful but also full of skin-loving vitamins.

- **Healthy Fats:** Avocado toast isn't just Instagram-worthy. It's also packed with healthy fats that moisturize the skin from within.

- **Green Tea:** Rich in antioxidants and boasting anti-inflammatory properties, it's a skin super drink!

Limit or Reduce:

- **Sugar:** Excess sugar can break down collagen. Time to rethink that second slice of cake!

- **Excess Dairy:** Some people may find dairy triggers breakouts. If you suspect it, maybe try reducing it and see how your skin responds.

- **Processed Foods:** They might be quick and tasty, but they lack the nutrients our skin so deeply desires.

4. Practical Skin-loving Exercise Tips

Hydrate Before and After:
Ensure you're well-hydrated before working out. It helps

regulate body temperature and replenish any fluid lost during the session.

Mind the Sun:
Outdoor exercises are refreshing, but remember to apply sunscreen. And if you're swimming, a waterproof one is a must.

Stretching:
It helps in toning the skin, improving elasticity, and delivering that radiant glow. So, before you wrap up, stretch it out!

5. Sync with Your Skin's Cycle

Our skin has its rhythms. During the day, it's all about protection. So, foods rich in antioxidants and applying sunscreen can be your best bet. Nighttime is when the skin repairs and regenerates. Omega-3s, zinc, and protein-rich foods can be ideal.

6. The Microbiome and Your Skin

Hey, have you heard of the term 'microbiome' before? No, it's not a new skincare brand. It's the community of tiny organisms, including bacteria, fungi, and viruses, that live on our skin. Don't squirm! These microorganisms are our friends. They play a crucial role in ensuring our skin remains healthy and radiant.

Fermented Foods:
Your daily dose of yogurt, kimchi, or kombucha does more than just aiding digestion. These probiotic-rich foods help maintain a balanced skin microbiome, keeping pesky breakouts at bay.

Prebiotics:
Think of these as food for your friendly skin bacteria. Foods like garlic, onions, and asparagus fuel the beneficial

bacteria on our skin, ensuring it remains balanced and healthy.

7. The Importance of Sleep

There's a reason it's called "beauty sleep." When we sleep, our body gets busy with repair and regeneration, including our skin. Deep, restful sleep ensures that our skin has ample time to recover from daily stressors.

Chamomile Tea:
This calming beverage can help induce sleep, ensuring your skin gets the restorative time it needs.

Limiting Caffeine and Sugar:
For that radiant morning glow, limit caffeine and sugar intake, especially in the evenings. They can disrupt sleep patterns, robbing your skin of its much-needed rest.

8. Skincare Rituals - Not Just Vanity

A skincare routine is more than just a self-vanity project. It's self-love. Cleansing, toning, and moisturizing can become meditative rituals, allowing us some 'me' time in our hectic lives.

Double Cleansing:
Popularized by Korean skincare routines, this involves using an oil-based cleanser followed by a water-based one. It ensures your skin is squeaky clean, free from pollutants and makeup.

Facial Massages:
Investing in a jade roller or simply using your fingers can boost blood circulation, giving your skin a natural, healthy tint.

9. Your Environment and Your Skin

Our surroundings profoundly affect our skin. Pollution, hard water, or even the air conditioning can strip our skin of its natural oils.

Indoor Plants:
Did you know that certain indoor plants can purify the air? Spider plants and snake plants are not only easy to maintain but also help in reducing indoor pollutants.

Humidifiers:
If you're in a dry environment, consider investing in a humidifier. It ensures the air remains moist, preventing your skin from drying out.

In this beautiful journey of life, our skin narrates our tales - from the laughter lines that showcase our happiest moments to the tiny scars that remind us of our adventures. It's not about striving for perfection but embracing and nourishing what we have. Remember, a happy skin is a reflection of a healthy inside. So, here's to celebrating the skin we're in, with the right foods, movement, and a whole lot of love!

19 DETOX AND CLEAN LIVING: SAFEGUARDING HEALTH IN A POLLUTED WORLD

Introduction

Hey there, Superwoman!

In today's world, environmental pollution is a reality that we all face. Air pollution, water contaminants, and exposure to various chemicals in our daily lives can potentially have adverse effects on our health. This is where the concept of detoxification and clean living comes into play.

Our bodies have a natural detoxification system primarily centered in the liver, kidneys, and digestive system. These organs work to process and eliminate toxins from our bodies. However, with the increasing burden of environmental toxins, supporting this natural detox process has become more crucial than ever.

Eating a diet rich in antioxidants and nutrients can help support your body's natural detox processes. Foods like leafy greens, berries, garlic, and cruciferous vegetables like broccoli and cauliflower are excellent choices. These foods provide essential vitamins and minerals that aid in detoxification.

Drinking plenty of clean, filtered water is essential for flushing out toxins and supporting kidney function. Staying hydrated is a fundamental aspect of detoxification.

Clean living also involves being mindful of the products you use in your daily life. Opt for natural, chemical-free cleaning products, skincare items, and cosmetics whenever possible. Reducing exposure to harmful chemicals can make a significant difference.

Regular exercise stimulates circulation and supports the lymphatic system, which plays a role in detoxifying the body. Sweating during exercise also helps eliminate toxins through the skin.

Chronic stress can hinder detoxification. Engaging in stress-reduction practices like meditation, deep breathing, or yoga can help your body detox more effectively.

Quality sleep is when your body does much of its repair and detoxification work. Ensure you get enough restful sleep to support these essential processes.

Reducing alcohol consumption and minimizing processed foods, which often contain additives and preservatives, can reduce the toxin load on your body.

If you're considering a more intensive detox program, it's advisable to consult a healthcare provider or a qualified nutritionist. They can provide guidance tailored to your specific needs and health goals.

In between juggling work, family, friends, and perhaps that weekly yoga class, have you ever felt like our fast-paced, modern world is taking a toll on your health? From the air we breathe to the water we drink, it seems like toxins are everywhere. But fear not! This chapter is going to be your roadmap for navigating through the haze of pollution and steering towards a cleaner, healthier life. Let's deep dive into the world of detox and clean living, shall we?

1. Understanding Detox: Myth vs. Reality

Okay, so let's get something straight - detoxing doesn't mean starving yourself or solely sipping on green juices for days on end. Your body has natural detoxification processes, primarily through the liver, kidneys, and even the skin. The key is to support and enhance these processes.

The Myth of "Detox Diets":
Heard of that latest '10-day detox' fad diet? Be wary. Often, these diets are restrictive and lack scientific backing. True detox is about supporting your body, not punishing it.

2. Clean Eating: Nature's Own Detox

"Let food be thy medicine," they say. And they're right! Mother Nature has blessed us with a plethora of foods that naturally help in detoxification.

Cruciferous Veggies:
Broccoli, cauliflower, and Brussels sprouts contain compounds that help the liver neutralize toxic substances.

Beets:
These vibrant roots support our liver, ensuring it functions optimally.

Citrus Fruits:
Lemons, oranges, and grapefruits are rich in antioxidants and help rejuvenate our bodies.

3. The Water Factor

Water isn't just essential for survival; it's our body's primary detox agent.

Stay Hydrated:
Drinking ample water ensures toxins are flushed out through urine.

Consider Filters:
With the rise in water pollution, consider investing in a good water filter. It'll ensure you're sipping on clean, contaminant-free water.

4. Breathe Clean

Did you know that indoor air can often be more polluted than outdoor air? Shocking, right?

House Plants to the Rescue:
Plants like peace lilies and spider plants act as natural air purifiers.

Air Purifiers:
For those living in urban areas, an air purifier can be a lifesaver, especially during times of high pollution.

5. Mindful Consumerism

Let's chat about that shopping spree. Sometimes, the toxins we need to be wary of are in the products we willingly bring into our homes.

Go Organic:
Pesticide residue on fruits and vegetables can be harmful. Opting for organic produce can be a cleaner choice.

Read Labels:
Whether it's your favorite lipstick or that new cleaning spray, understanding ingredient lists can help you make healthier choices.

6. Embrace Nature: The Ultimate Detox

Taking a break and connecting with nature can be incredibly detoxifying for the mind and soul.

Forest Bathing:
The Japanese practice of 'Shinrin-Yoku' involves taking in the forest atmosphere. It's been shown to lower stress hormone production, improve feelings of happiness, and free up creativity!

7. Digital Detox

In a digitally connected world, sometimes the most toxic elements are intangible.

Screen Breaks:
Make it a habit to take frequent screen breaks. Your eyes and mind will thank you.

Unplugging Rituals:
Choose a day or a few hours in the week to completely unplug. Read a book, take a walk, or simply meditate.

8. Say No to Processed Foods

In the hustle and bustle of daily life, grabbing that pack of instant noodles or microwaving ready-to-eat meals might seem convenient. But here's the thing:

Hidden Culprits: Processed foods often contain preservatives, artificial colors, and trans fats. These aren't friends to your body. Over time, they accumulate and can affect your liver and overall health.

Make It Fresh: Take some time out each week to plan your meals. Opt for fresh salads, wholesome grains, and homemade curries or stir-fries. Your body will reward you with increased energy and vitality.

9. Reduce Alcohol and Caffeine

I know, I know, that glass of wine after a hectic day or the morning cuppa joe feels oh-so-right. But moderation is key!

Love for the Liver: Excessive alcohol can strain the liver, the organ primarily responsible for detoxifying your body. So, go easy on the cocktails and beers.

Caffeine Check: While coffee has its health benefits, overconsumption can dehydrate and may interfere with sleep. And a rested body is a detoxified body.

10. Skin: Your Detoxifying Organ

That's right! Our skin isn't just there to make us look good; it plays a crucial role in detoxification.

Dry Brushing: An age-old technique that involves brushing your skin with natural bristles to stimulate circulation and slough off dead skin cells. It's like giving your skin a mini detox session.

Sweat It Out: Whether it's through a workout, a sauna, or even a spicy meal, sweating helps release toxins. So, let those pores breathe!

11. The Magic of Herbal Teas

There's a herbal tea for almost every health concern, and detoxification is no exception.

Dandelion Tea: Supports liver function and has a mildly diuretic effect, helping you eliminate toxins faster.

Green Tea: Rich in antioxidants, it not only aids detoxification but also boosts metabolism.

12. Mindful Movement: Detox through Exercise

You might think, "How does exercise relate to detox?" But trust me, it's all connected.

Boosted Circulation: Regular movement helps increase blood circulation, ensuring that nutrients reach every cell and waste products are efficiently removed.

Deep Breathing: Ever noticed those deep breaths during yoga or pilates? Deep breathing helps in better oxygen exchange, playing a role in releasing toxins.

13. Mental Detox: It's Real

Detox isn't just physical. Our mind, with its myriad thoughts, needs a cleanse too.

Meditation and Mindfulness: Taking a few minutes daily to meditate can help in decluttering the mind.

Limit Negativity: Whether it's news, toxic relationships, or self-deprecating thoughts, limiting negativity can have a profound impact on mental well-being.

Conclusion

My dear readers, detoxification is a holistic process. It's not just about what you eat or drink, but also about the environment you create both externally and internally. It's about making informed choices and recognizing the subtle signals our bodies send us. And remember, while the world may be filled with pollutants, you have the power and knowledge to rise above and live a cleaner, more vibrant life. Let's make every day a detox day! Here's to living pure in an impure world. Cheers to your health!

20 MINDFUL MOVEMENT: THE MENTAL BENEFITS OF PHYSICAL ACTIVITY

Hello dear reader!

Remember the days when you felt all cooped up and restless, and then you took a walk and suddenly everything felt better? Or maybe you've had days where you couldn't quite shake off that cloud of gloom until you did some yoga or danced around your living room? There's a reason for that - movement is not just about the body. It's intricately linked to our minds.

1. Setting the Scene: The Mind-Body Connection

Hey, did you know that our minds and bodies are not separate entities? Instead, they function as a beautifully intertwined duo. The ancient Greeks believed in the philosophy of "a sound mind in a sound body." Think about it: ever felt butterflies in your stomach when nervous or a weight on your shoulders when stressed? That's the mind-body connection right there.

2. The Endorphin Rush: It's Real and It's Fabulous

Remember that 'high' you feel after a jog or a rigorous Zumba session? Meet endorphins - our body's natural mood elevators. Physical activity stimulates the release of these happy chemicals. They're nature's way of telling you, "Hey, thanks for moving me!"

3. Stress Buster 101: Say Hello to Reduced Cortisol

Cortisol – sounds like a fancy name, right? It's the body's primary stress hormone. While necessary in certain situations (like when you need to flee from danger), chronic high levels can be detrimental. Exercise helps regulate cortisol, ensuring you don't remain in a perpetual "fight or flight" mode.

4. Yoga and Mindfulness: The Dynamic Duo

Yoga isn't just about getting those Instagram-worthy poses. The deep breaths, the stretches, the holding of poses - they're all grounding experiences. They teach patience, resilience, and focus. And did I mention the relaxation at the end, during 'Savasana'? Pure bliss!

5. Dancing: Joy, Freedom, and a Dash of Nostalgia

Dance like no one's watching. Why? Because it's liberating! Dancing isn't just about the steps; it's about expressing feelings and emotions. It takes you back to simpler times, to childhood days, and brings forth uninhibited joy.

6. Movement as Meditation: The Zen of Repetition

Activities like Tai Chi, Qi Gong, or even just regular walking can be meditative. The repetitive movements, combined with focused breathing, bring about a tranquility that's hard to beat. It's like your body finds its rhythm, and the mind just chimes in.

7. Boosting Brain Power: The Cognitive Benefits

Research shows that regular physical activity can improve cognitive functions. Remember the old saying, "All work and no play makes Jack a dull boy?" It's scientifically true! Movement can boost memory, alertness, and even creativity.

8. Social Butterflies: Group Activities and Mental Well-being

Joining a dance class, group hikes, or even weekly jogging clubs can enhance social connections. And as humans, we're wired for connection. It offers a sense of belonging, reduces feelings of loneliness, and boosts our overall mental health.

9. Reconnecting with Nature: The Outdoors as a Therapist

Nature walks, treks, or even a simple jog in the park – being outdoors and among nature has its own set of mental benefits. The greenery, the chirping birds, the gentle breeze – they don't just soothe the soul; they rejuvenate the mind.

10. A Note on Rest: The Importance of Recovery

Now, here's a twist. Movement is essential, yes, but so is rest. The quiet moments post-exercise, the days you let your body recover – they are as crucial as the activity itself. It's in these silent intervals that the body heals, and the mind reflects.

Mindful movement is the practice of combining physical activity with a heightened sense of awareness and presence. It's about being fully engaged in the activity you're doing, whether it's yoga, walking, dancing, or any form of exercise.

The Mental Benefits of Mindful Movement:

Stress Reduction: Mindful movement is a powerful stress reducer. When you're fully present in the moment, it's challenging for stressors to dominate your thoughts. This can lead to reduced feelings of anxiety and a greater sense of calm.

Improved Mood: Physical activity releases endorphins, those feel-good hormones that can elevate your mood. When combined with mindfulness, it's like a double dose of positivity for your brain.

Enhanced Mental Clarity: Engaging in mindful movement can improve your mental focus and clarity. It's almost like a mini-meditation session where you clear your mind of clutter and gain mental sharpness.

Emotional Regulation: Mindful movement encourages emotional awareness. You become more attuned to your emotions, allowing you to manage them better. This can be particularly helpful for those dealing with mood disorders.

Better Body Image: By focusing on the sensations and movements of your body rather than its appearance, mindful movement can promote a healthier body image and self-esteem.

Increased Resilience: Regular mindful movement can build mental resilience. It teaches you to stay present even in challenging situations, which can translate into better coping skills in daily life.

Social Connection: Many mindful movement practices, like group fitness classes or team sports, foster a sense of community and social connection. Social support is crucial for mental well-being.

Tips for Mindful Movement:

Start Slow: If you're new to mindful movement, begin with short sessions and gradually build up. The key is consistency.

Breathe: Pay attention to your breath as you move. Deep, rhythmic breathing enhances the mindfulness experience.

Sensory Awareness: Focus on the sensations in your body —the feeling of your feet hitting the ground, the stretch in your muscles, the rhythm of your heartbeat.

Stay Present: When your mind wanders (as it inevitably will), gently bring your focus back to the present moment and the movement you're doing.

Variety: Explore different forms of mindful movement to find what resonates with you. It could be yoga, tai chi, hiking, or even mindful walking.

Conclusion:

Dear reader, movement isn't merely about sculpting muscles or achieving fitness milestones. It's therapy, meditation, joy, and so much more rolled into one. It's about celebrating what our bodies can do and cherishing the mental tranquility that follows. So, the next time you're feeling low or stressed, remember that movement can be your refuge. Here's to mindful movement and the beauty of the mind-body symphony.

21 ANCIENT WISDOM AND MODERN SCIENCE: INTEGRATING TRADITIONAL AND CONTEMPORARY APPROACHES

Hey there, lovely reader!

Have you ever been intrigued by the allure of ancient practices? The aromatic herbs of Ayurveda, the flowing movements of Tai Chi, or the focused tranquility of meditation? But then again, we can't ignore the groundbreaking advancements of modern science either. What if we didn't have to choose? What if we could blend the best of both worlds?

1. A Timeless Journey: Embracing the Old and the New

Once upon a time, our ancestors relied on the rhythms of nature, the phases of the moon, and the herbs in their backyard. They were deeply connected to the world around them. Fast forward to today, we have technology, data, and a myriad of scientific tools at our disposal. The beauty? Both can coexist, and when they do, magic happens!

2. The Ayurvedic Chronicle: Your Dosha and Modern Nutrition

Ayurveda, an ancient Indian medicinal practice, is all about balance. It categorizes us into different 'doshas' or body types. Guess what? Modern nutritional science often aligns with these age-old principles, only with fancy terms like 'metabolic types' or 'bio-individuality'.

3. Acupuncture Meets Neuroscience

Those tiny needles aren't just for show! Traditional Chinese medicine has used acupuncture for centuries to channel the body's energy or 'chi'. Modern neuroscience says, "Hey, they might be onto something!" by showing us how acupuncture points align with nerve endings and can influence neurotransmitter release.

4. Herbal Remedies: From Grandma's Backyard to the Modern Lab

Remember grandma's turmeric milk for colds or the ginger tea for digestion? Modern pharmacology is now isolating active compounds from these herbs, understanding their mechanisms, and even integrating them into mainstream medicine. It's like the past shaking hands with the present!

5. Yoga and Physiotherapy: Stretching Across Time

Those yoga stretches aren't just spiritual; they're also physiological wonders. Modern physiotherapy often incorporates age-old yoga postures, acknowledging their benefits for musculoskeletal health. The ancient yogis sure knew their anatomy!

6. Meditation and Mindfulness in the Age of MRIs

Once considered a purely spiritual endeavor, meditation is now under the scanner—quite literally. Modern MRI machines showcase the positive brain changes brought about by consistent meditation practices. It's not just about inner peace; it's about neuroplasticity.

7. The Ancient Art of Fasting and Modern Intermittent Fasting

Fasting has been around for ages, embedded in various cultural and religious practices. Today, intermittent fasting is a buzzword in the health and fitness community. Science says it can boost metabolism, promote longevity, and even improve cognitive function. Our ancestors? They probably just called it "routine."

8. Plant-Based Diets: Wisdom of the Ancients, Endorsed by Science

Long before it was trendy, many ancient cultures were primarily plant-based due to both health and spiritual reasons. Modern nutritional science now highlights the myriad benefits of such diets, from cardiovascular health to reduced cancer risks.

9. Balneotherapy and Modern Spa Treatments

The ancient Romans loved their baths. They believed in the therapeutic properties of water. Cut to modern-day spa treatments, and we see a blend of age-old balneotherapy practices with contemporary knowledge. Water isn't just for hydration; it's for healing.

Ancient Wisdom on Food:

Throughout history, various cultures have developed profound wisdom when it comes to food and nutrition. Here are some key highlights:

1. Ayurveda in India: Dating back thousands of years, Ayurveda is one of the world's oldest holistic healing systems. It emphasizes a personalized approach to diet based on an individual's constitution, known as doshas. This ancient wisdom encourages balance in food choices to promote health and well-being.

2. Chinese Medicine: Traditional Chinese Medicine (TCM) is another ancient system that places great importance on food. It classifies foods into categories such as cooling or warming and believes that the balance of these properties in one's diet can impact health. TCM also emphasizes the concept of Qi, the vital life force, and how food can either strengthen or weaken it.

3. Mediterranean Diet: The Mediterranean region has a long history of dietary wisdom. The Mediterranean diet, characterized by abundant fruits, vegetables, whole grains, olive oil, and moderate consumption of wine and lean protein, has been linked to lower rates of heart disease and longer life spans.

4. Japanese Cuisine: Japan's traditional diet, rich in seafood, vegetables, and fermented foods like miso and soy sauce, is known for its health benefits. It's credited with contributing to the longevity of the Japanese population.

5. Native American Wisdom: Native American cultures have deep-rooted knowledge of indigenous plants and sustainable farming practices. Their traditional diets often consisted of locally sourced, whole foods that were not only nourishing but also respectful of the environment.

Ancient Wisdom on Physical Activity:

Physical activity has always been an integral part of human history, often intertwined with cultural and practical aspects of life. Here's a glimpse of ancient wisdom related to physical activity:

1. Ancient Greece: In ancient Greece, physical activity was highly valued and integrated into daily life. The Greek philosophers, including Aristotle and Hippocrates, recognized the importance of exercise for maintaining health and balance. The Olympic Games, originating in Greece, were a celebration of physical prowess.

2. Yoga and India: Yoga, with roots dating back over 5,000 years, is a prime example of ancient wisdom in physical activity. It combines postures, breathing techniques, and meditation to promote physical and mental well-being. Yoga is a testament to the belief that movement is not just about fitness but also inner harmony.

3. Martial Arts in Asia: Asian cultures developed a range of martial arts, such as karate, kung fu, and judo. These practices not only taught self-defense but also promoted discipline, mental focus, and physical fitness. They emphasized the connection between mind and body.

4. Indigenous Movement: Indigenous cultures around the world have practiced traditional dances, hunting, and gathering activities that are both physically demanding and culturally significant. These activities have preserved their physical and mental health for generations.

5. Roman Engineering: The Romans understood the importance of physical activity for their soldiers' readiness. They built extensive systems of aqueducts, roads, and arenas, which enabled the practice of various physical activities, including bathing, running, and combat training.

The Modern Connection:

What's striking is how much of this ancient wisdom on food and activity aligns with modern scientific findings. Concepts like balance, whole foods, mindfulness, and the importance of physical activity for both physical and mental health are as relevant today as they were centuries ago.

In many ways, modern science is rediscovering and validating the wisdom of our ancestors. It's an exciting time where ancient traditions and modern research can complement each other to guide us toward healthier, more balanced lives.

So, as we explore the history of ancient wisdom on food and activity, we find that the lessons from our ancestors continue to be valuable guides on our journey to well-being, reminding us that the keys to a healthy life have deep and enduring roots in our shared human history.

Conclusion:

Dear reader, isn't it fascinating how the spirals of time converge? How ancient wisdom, often passed down through stories and traditions, finds validation in the gleaming halls of modern labs? As we step into the future, let's carry the treasures of the past with us. For in this marriage of the ancient and the contemporary, we find holistic health and true well-being. Cheers to blending the old with the new!

22 PERSONALISED NUTRITION: CRAFTING A DIET THAT'S RIGHT FOR YOU

Hey there, beautiful soul! ✨

You know how they say, "One man's food is another man's poison"? Well, there's more truth to that than you might think. In the age of Instagram-worthy avocado toasts and green smoothies, it can feel like there's a "perfect diet" everyone but you is following. But here's the tea: there isn't one.

Why? Because each one of us is unique – from our DNA to our lifestyle, and our gut bacteria to our taste buds. Let's dive deep and see how you can craft a diet that celebrates YOU.

1. The Puzzle of Personalization

Remember when you tried that keto diet your colleague raved about but felt exhausted? Or when you ate like your fitness-idol but just didn't get the same results? It's not about what works; it's about what works *for you*.

2. Genes and Jeans: DNA-Based Diets

Science alert! 🧬 Ever heard of nutrigenomics? It's the study of how our genes interact with our diet. By understanding our genetic makeup, we can predict how we might respond to certain foods. Imagine knowing that your body thrives on a Mediterranean diet or that you're lactose intolerant just by scanning your genes!

3. The Marvelous World Within: Your Gut Microbiome

Our gut houses trillions of bacteria, and no two guts are identical. They play a role in digesting food, making vitamins, and even influencing our mood. The state of our microbiome can guide our food choices. More fermented foods? Less sugar? Your gut bugs have an opinion!

4. Blood Type Diets: Fact or Fiction?

Some say that our blood type should dictate our diet. O types should go paleo, A types vegetarian...but what does science say? Let's dissect this popular diet theory together.

5. Ayurveda and Personalized Nutrition

Coming from ancient India, Ayurveda classifies us into 'doshas' based on our body type and personality. It's fascinating how this age-old wisdom can guide our modern plates.

6. Tapping into Intuitive Eating

Beyond genes and gut bacteria, there's another guide: your intuition. Learning to listen to your body's cues – hunger, fullness, cravings – is a journey in self-awareness and trust. Let's explore how to tune in.

7. Activity Levels and Appetites

Athletes need a different diet than sedentary individuals. A yoga instructor's needs differ from a marathon runner's. How active are you, and what does that mean for your plate?

8. Life Stages and Nutritional Needs

From the growing needs of teens, the nutritional demands of pregnancy, to the changing landscape of menopause – our diet should evolve as we dance through different life stages.

9. Crafting Your Personal Diet: Practical Steps

Ready to be your nutritionist? Here's a roadmap to craft a diet that's tailored just for you. From food journaling, genetic testing, consulting with professionals, to simply checking in with yourself – we've got you covered.

Some real-world use cases to illustrate how it can benefit individuals.

Use Case 1: Weight Management

Meet Sarah, a 35-year-old woman struggling with weight management. She's tried various diets, but nothing seems to work. With personalized nutrition:

- **Genetic Insights:** Sarah undergoes genetic testing, which reveals that she has a genetic predisposition to insulin resistance. This information guides her diet plan to focus on low-glycemic foods, helping stabilize her blood sugar levels.

- **Lifestyle Assessment:** Sarah's personalized plan takes her busy work schedule into account. It includes quick, healthy meal options and snack ideas that fit her on-the-go lifestyle.

- **Health Goals:** Sarah's primary goal is weight loss and improved overall health. Her personalized plan incorporates portion control, a balanced macronutrient ratio, and regular exercise recommendations tailored to her fitness level.

Result: Sarah experiences steady weight loss and increased energy. The personalized approach addresses her unique challenges and keeps her motivated.

Use Case 2: Managing a Chronic Condition

John is a 45-year-old man recently diagnosed with hypertension (high blood pressure). He's concerned about his health and wants to manage his condition effectively. With personalized nutrition:

- **Genetic Insights:** Genetic testing reveals that John has a genetic predisposition to salt sensitivity. His personalized plan includes a lower-sodium diet tailored to his preferences.

- **Lifestyle Assessment:** John's busy job and sedentary lifestyle are taken into account. His plan includes simple, home-cooked meals that are easy to prepare and regular reminders for short breaks to move and stretch during work hours.

- **Health Goals:** John's primary goal is to manage his blood pressure and reduce his risk of heart disease. His personalized plan emphasizes heart-healthy foods like leafy greens, lean proteins, and potassium-rich fruits.

Result: John's blood pressure gradually decreases, and he learns to make sustainable, heart-healthy choices that improve his overall well-being.

Use Case 3: Athletic Performance

Alex is a competitive cyclist aiming to enhance his athletic performance. He's looking to fine-tune his nutrition for better results. With personalized nutrition:

- **Genetic Insights:** Genetic testing reveals that Alex has a variant associated with a higher need for carbohydrates during endurance exercise. His personalized plan includes carb-loading strategies before races.

- **Lifestyle Assessment:** Alex's demanding training schedule requires careful fueling. His plan includes precise timing for pre-workout and post-workout meals and snacks, optimizing his energy levels and recovery.

- **Health Goals:** Alex's primary goal is peak performance. His personalized plan ensures he meets his calorie and nutrient needs to support his intense training regimen.

Result: Alex experiences improved endurance, faster recovery, and better race results, thanks to his personalized nutrition plan.

Use Case 4: Allergy Management

Meet Emily, a 28-year-old woman who has struggled with food allergies for most of her life. She's determined to find a way to enjoy a diverse diet safely. With personalized nutrition:

- **Genetic Insights:** Emily's genetic testing reveals that she has a genetic predisposition to certain food allergies. This information helps her healthcare provider craft a diet plan that avoids trigger foods while ensuring she gets all the necessary nutrients.

- **Lifestyle Assessment:** Emily's busy schedule doesn't leave much time for extensive food preparation. Her personalized plan includes quick and easy allergy-safe recipes and a list of allergy-friendly restaurants in her area.

- **Health Goals:** Emily's primary goal is to manage her allergies and enjoy a varied and nutritious diet. Her personalized plan emphasizes allergy-safe substitutes and creative meal ideas to keep her meals interesting.

Result: Emily discovers a wide range of delicious allergy-friendly foods and enjoys a healthier, more balanced diet while safely managing her allergies.

Use Case 5: Nutritional Support During Pregnancy

Sophia is a soon-to-be mother, and she wants to ensure a healthy pregnancy for both herself and her baby. With personalized nutrition:

- **Genetic Insights:** Genetic testing reveals that Sophia has a genetic predisposition to vitamin D deficiency. Her personalized plan includes vitamin D-rich foods and supplements to support her pregnancy.

- **Lifestyle Assessment:** Sophia's busy lifestyle and pregnancy-induced fatigue are taken into account. Her plan includes simple and nutritious meal ideas that cater to her energy levels and changing cravings.

- **Health Goals:** Sophia's primary goal is a healthy pregnancy and the well-being of her baby. Her personalized plan focuses on foods rich in folate, iron, calcium, and other essential nutrients required during pregnancy.

Result: Sophia experiences a healthy pregnancy with adequate nutrient intake, supporting both her and her baby's well-being.

These use cases illustrate how personalized nutrition can address a wide range of individual health needs and goals, from managing allergies and supporting pregnancy to enhancing athletic performance and addressing chronic conditions. By tailoring dietary recommendations to each person's unique characteristics, personalized nutrition empowers individuals to make informed choices that support their well-being and health objectives.

Conclusion:

Hey superstar, remember: in the world of nutrition, one size doesn't fit all. And that's a good thing! It means there's a unique path, carved out just for you, waiting to be discovered. Embrace the journey, celebrate the discoveries, and remember to savor every bite. Your perfect diet isn't the one in a best-selling book; it's the one that makes you feel alive, vibrant, and utterly YOU.

Till our next heart-to-heart, keep shining and eating joyfully!

23 EMBRACING CHANGE: ADAPTING TO LIFE'S DIFFERENT PHASES

Hello, radiant soul!

Life is an ever-revolving door of change, isn't it? Just when we think we've got things figured out – BOOM! – a curveball comes our way. Be it the roller coaster of puberty, the transformative years of adulthood, or the graceful journey into the golden years, each phase comes with its own set of wonders and woes.

But here's the good news: embracing change can be beautiful, empowering, and, dare I say, fun! Ready to embark on this journey with me? Buckle up, and let's go!

1. The Tumultuous Teens: Puberty and Everything in Between

Remember those teenage years? Ah, the drama! The acne, the growth spurts, and the emotional roller coasters. The teenage body and mind are a whirlwind of hormonal changes. Let's revisit those years and uncover the beauty beneath the chaos.

2. The Roaring Twenties: Discovering Yourself

Oh, the twenties! A time of freedom, exploration, and yes, a few existential crises. Whether it's navigating relationships, kickstarting careers, or just figuring out who we are, this decade is chock-full of lessons and laughter.

3. The Thriving Thirties: Balancing Act

Often touted as the 'best years of our lives', the thirties can be a mixed bag. Juggling career, family, personal aspirations, and the ever-ticking biological clock – it's about mastering the art of balance. And guess what? You totally got this!

4. The Fabulous Forties: Reflection and Reinvention

Some call it the 'mid-life crisis', but I prefer 'mid-life awakening'. This decade is all about self-reflection, re-evaluation, and sometimes, a complete reinvention. It's the perfect time to ask: "Who have I become, and who do I want to be?"

5. The Fulfilling Fifties: Embracing Wisdom

With kids growing up and possibly flying the nest, the fifties can be a transformative period. It's a time of profound wisdom, a deeper understanding of oneself, and often, a rediscovery of passions that might have taken a backseat.

6. The Serene Sixties and Beyond: The Golden Era

Ah, the golden years! A time to bask in the glow of well-earned rest, to indulge in hobbies, and to spend quality time with loved ones. It's also a phase of introspection, acceptance, and profound peace.

7. Dealing with Change: Emotional and Mental Strategies

Change can be daunting, but it doesn't have to be. Equip yourself with emotional tools and mental strategies to dance gracefully through life's ever-changing rhythms.

8. The Physicality of Change: Body Adjustments

Our bodies evolve, and so should our self-care strategies. From skincare regimes to dietary adjustments, let's explore how to honor and care for our changing bodies.

9. Building Resilience through Life's Phases

Life can throw some tough punches. But with resilience, we can not only withstand challenges but thrive amidst them. Dive deep into the art and science of building a resilient spirit.

Stories

Story 1: "The Marathon Mom"

Meet Sarah, a mother of two in her mid-30s. She used to be a competitive runner in her youth but had to put her passion on hold to raise her kids. As her children grew older, Sarah decided it was time to embrace change and return to running. She realized she couldn't train like she used to due to her family and work commitments. Instead, she adapted by waking up early to run, involving her kids in her training, and finding local races that were family-friendly. Sarah didn't aim for personal records; instead, she focused on the joy of running and setting an example of an active, adaptable life for her children. Through these changes, she not only found her way back to the sport she loved but also inspired her family to lead healthier lives.

Story 2: "Graceful Aging"

James, a retired schoolteacher in his 70s, was experiencing the natural changes that come with aging. His mobility was decreasing, and he faced some health challenges. Rather than resisting these changes, he decided to embrace them. James enrolled in gentle yoga classes designed for seniors to improve his flexibility and balance. He adapted his diet to include more nutrient-rich foods, understanding the importance of bone health and cardiovascular well-being. James also joined a local seniors' group, where he formed new friendships and stayed socially engaged. His positive attitude and adaptability not only improved his health but also inspired those around him to age gracefully and make the most of their golden years.

Story 3: "The Career Transition"

Lisa had built a successful career in her 40s but was feeling unfulfilled and stressed. She longed for a change but was unsure of what to do next. After some soul-searching and exploring her passions, she decided to make a career transition. Lisa knew it wouldn't be easy, but she was determined to embrace this new phase of her life. She enrolled in courses to gain new skills and networked with professionals in her chosen field. It was challenging, and there were moments of doubt, but Lisa persevered. Her adaptability paid off, and she eventually found a fulfilling career in a completely different industry. Lisa's story reminds us that it's never too late to make a change and follow your dreams, even if it means starting over in a new phase of life.

These stories highlight how individuals from various phases of life have successfully embraced change and adapted to their evolving circumstances, leading to personal growth, well-being, and fulfillment. Embracing change is not always easy, but it can lead to incredible transformations and a more enriching life journey.

Conclusion:

Gorgeous soul, remember this: every phase of life is a chapter in the beautiful book that is YOU. Instead of fearing change, let's embrace it, celebrate it, and grow through it. Because at the end of the day, it's not about the years in our life but the life in our years.

Keep shining, keep evolving, and remember – life's best moments often come wrapped in the cloak of change.

Until our next heart-to-heart, stay radiant!

24 BUILDING A SUPPORTIVE COMMUNITY: THE ROLE OF SOCIAL CONNECTIONS IN HEALTH

Hey there, amazing human!

You know, it often amazes me how we can have hundreds of "friends" on social media, yet sometimes feel so alone in the offline world. It's a paradox of our times, isn't it? Yet deep down, we all know that real-life, genuine connections are vital for our well-being. They're like the sunshine to our blooming flower, the peanut butter to our jelly. Let's deep dive into why and how these connections truly nourish our soul and health.

1. The Science of Social Connections

Let's get nerdy for a moment! Studies consistently show that strong social ties can boost our mental health, improve our immunity, and even increase our lifespan. Yes, having a supportive friend can indeed add years to your life!

2. Quality over Quantity: The Depth of Connections

It's not about having a crowd around you; it's about having those few who truly understand your heart's song. Let's chat about why deep, meaningful relationships outshine a plethora of surface-level ones.

3. Building Your Tribe: Where and How to Find Your People

Whether you're an extrovert, introvert, or somewhere in between (hello, ambiverts!), there are ways and places to find your tribe. From hobby clubs to volunteering, let's explore avenues to find those soul connections.

4. Nurturing the Bonds: Keeping Relationships Alive and Thriving

Relationships, like plants, need nurturing. Whether it's setting boundaries, expressing gratitude, or simply showing up – delve into the art of relationship maintenance.

5. The Digital Age: Online Communities and Their Value

In our tech-driven world, online communities can offer immense value. From support groups to forums dedicated to specific interests, let's uncover the beauty of virtual camaraderie.

6. When Bonds Break: Navigating Relationship Strains and Endings

Ouch. This one's a bit sensitive, isn't it? Not all relationships last forever, and that's okay. Learn how to navigate these waters without drowning in sorrow and finding lessons amidst the pain.

7. Beyond Friends: The Role of Pets in Mental Well-being

Whoever said diamonds are a girl's best friend never had a pet! 🐾 Whether it's a wagging tail, a purring kitty, or a chirping bird, our furry (or feathery) friends offer invaluable emotional support.

8. Community Building Activities: Strengthening the Group Dynamic

Got a group of amazing people? Fantastic! Let's look at activities and ideas to strengthen the bond, foster trust, and create a reservoir of memories.

9. The Health Benefits of Group Activities

Whether it's a group yoga session, a community garden project, or a collective meditation – group activities have a unique charm and a plethora of health benefits. Let's explore!

Use Case 1: Seniors' Social Club

Problem: Grace, an 80-year-old widow, was struggling with loneliness and isolation due to living alone.

Meet Grace, an 80-year-old widow living alone. She was experiencing feelings of loneliness and isolation. A friend recommended she join a local seniors' social club. There, she found a supportive community of peers who shared stories, played games, and enjoyed activities together. Grace's regular interactions with the club members not only lifted her spirits but also improved her cognitive function and overall well-being. The social connections she formed at the club became an essential part of her life, helping her age gracefully and happily.

Solution: Joining a local seniors' social club provided Grace with a supportive community of peers. Regular interactions with club members alleviated her feelings of isolation and improved her cognitive function and overall well-being.

Use Case 2: Weight Loss Support Group

Problem: John had been battling obesity for years and needed support to make a lasting change.

John had struggled with obesity for years and decided it was time to make a change. He joined a weight loss support group in his community. Being part of a group that understood his challenges and goals provided him with valuable emotional support. The group shared healthy recipes, exercise tips, and celebrated each other's successes. With the encouragement of his new community, John lost weight, improved his health, and gained lifelong friends who continued to support his journey.

Solution: Joining a weight loss support group allowed John to connect with others facing similar challenges. This supportive community shared tips, celebrated successes, and provided emotional encouragement, ultimately helping him lose weight and gain lifelong friends who continued to support his journey.

Use Case 3: Pandemic Virtual Support Network

Problem: Sarah, a young professional working from home, felt socially isolated during the COVID-19 pandemic due to lockdowns and restrictions.

During the COVID-19 pandemic, many people experienced social isolation due to lockdowns and restrictions. Sarah, a young professional working from home, found it challenging to cope with the sudden lack of social interactions. She joined a virtual support network organized by her workplace. Through video calls and online chats, she connected with colleagues facing similar challenges. Sharing their experiences and strategies for managing remote work helped alleviate her feelings of isolation and anxiety. The virtual community not only provided a sense of belonging but also contributed to her mental and emotional well-being during the challenging times.

Solution: Sarah found solace in a virtual support network organized by her workplace. Through video calls and online chats, she connected with colleagues facing similar challenges, reducing her feelings of isolation and anxiety. This virtual community not only provided a sense of belonging but also contributed to her mental and emotional well-being during challenging times.

Use Case 4: Community Garden

Problem: A bustling urban neighborhood lacked green spaces and opportunities for residents to connect.

In a bustling urban neighborhood, residents decided to transform an abandoned lot into a community garden. Neighbors of all ages came together to cultivate the garden, sharing their love for gardening and fresh produce. The garden not only provided a source of nutritious food but also became a hub for social interaction. Families, retirees, and young professionals bonded over shared tasks, exchanged gardening tips, and organized community events. The garden strengthened the neighborhood's sense of community and improved both physical and mental well-being.

Solution: Transforming an abandoned lot into a community garden brought neighbors together. This communal project not only provided nutritious food but also fostered social interaction, offering a sense of community and improving residents' physical and mental well-being.

Use Case 5: Online Health Support Group

Problem: Mark was diagnosed with a rare chronic illness and felt isolated and overwhelmed.

Mark was diagnosed with a rare chronic illness that left him feeling isolated and overwhelmed. He found solace in an online health support group dedicated to his condition. The group offered a safe space to discuss symptoms, treatments, and coping strategies. Mark gained valuable insights from others' experiences and felt emotionally supported by the group members. Over time, he not only managed his condition better but also formed lasting friendships with people who understood the challenges he faced.

Solution: Mark found solace in an online health support group dedicated to his condition. This virtual community provided a safe space to discuss symptoms, treatments, and coping strategies. It allowed him to gain valuable insights from others' experiences and receive emotional support, resulting in better management of his condition and lasting friendships with those who understood his challenges.

These use cases demonstrate how social connections and supportive communities can have a profound impact on individuals' physical and mental health. Whether in-person or virtual, these connections provide emotional support, motivation, and a sense of belonging that contribute significantly to overall well-being and quality of life.

Conclusion:

My dear friend, we're social beings. Our hearts thrive on connection, understanding, and mutual support. In the grand tapestry of life, these connections form the threads that make our experiences richer, our lows bearable, and our highs even more exhilarating.

So, reach out, build bridges, mend fences, and cherish the incredible humans around you. Because in the end, it's these bonds that add color, warmth, and profound meaning to our journey on this blue dot in the vast cosmos.

Until our next heartful conversation, keep connecting, keep loving!

25. FUELING YOUR AMBITIONS: NUTRITION AND EXERCISE FOR HIGH-ACHIEVERS

Hello, unstoppable go-getter!

You're the kind of person who dreams big, sets goals higher than skyscrapers, and thrives on challenges. But here's the deal: reaching those summits requires a different kind of fuel. It's like your life is a high-performance race car, and you need the premium-grade gas and top-notch mechanics to keep it running at its best. Let's dive into how the right nutrition and exercise can supercharge your ambitions.

1. High-Achievers Need High-Octane Fuel

Just like a luxury car performs best with premium fuel, your body operates optimally with the right nutrients. We'll talk about how your diet can match your ambition's intensity.

2. The Power of Nutrient Timing

Ever heard the phrase, "timing is everything"? That's true for nutrition too. We'll explore how eating at the right times can turbocharge your energy levels, focus, and overall productivity.

3. Stress Management for Superheroes

High-achievers often dance on the edge of stress. Let's uncover how nutrition and exercise can be your shields against burnout and your secret weapon for resilience.

4. Exercise as Brain Fuel

Exercise isn't just about looking good; it's about performing at your peak mentally. We'll discuss how workouts boost cognitive function, creativity, and problem-solving skills.

5. Superfoods for Super You

Certain foods are like rocket fuel for your body and mind. We'll create a list of these superfoods that can give you the edge in your high-stakes game.

6. The Art of Recovery

Pushing yourself to the limit? Recovery is where the magic happens. Learn how to optimize post-workout nutrition and sleep for faster, better results.

7. The High-Achiever's Workout Regimen

Your exercise routine should be as finely tuned as your daily schedule. We'll design a workout plan that maximizes your efficiency and effectiveness.

8. Mindful Movement: Yoga and Meditation for Peak Performance

Yoga and meditation aren't just for relaxation; they can enhance your focus, emotional intelligence, and decision-making abilities.

9. Balance for Longevity

Ambition without balance can lead to burnout. We'll discuss strategies for maintaining a fulfilling personal life alongside your professional pursuits.

Step-by-step guides for each of the five exercises mentioned:

1. Yoga:

Yoga is a versatile practice with various poses and styles. Here's a basic guide for a simple yoga routine:

- **Step 1:** Find a quiet, comfortable space where you won't be disturbed. Use a yoga mat or a soft surface.

- **Step 2:** Begin with deep breathing exercises to center yourself. Sit or lie down, close your eyes, and take slow, deep breaths in and out.

- **Step 3:** Start with basic poses like the Downward Dog, Child's Pose, or Cat-Cow Stretch. These poses help warm up your body and improve flexibility.

- **Step 4:** Progress to more challenging poses as you become comfortable with the basics. Poses like Warrior I and II, Tree Pose, and Cobra are great options.

- **Step 5:** Maintain a steady breath throughout your practice. Focus on mindfulness and being present in each pose.

- **Step 6:** End your practice with Savasana (Corpse Pose) for relaxation and reflection. Lie down on your mat, close your eyes, and let go of tension in your body.

2. High-Intensity Interval Training (HIIT):

HIIT workouts are short and intense. Here's a basic guide for a HIIT routine:

- **Step 1:** Warm up for 5-10 minutes with light cardio exercises like jumping jacks or jogging in place.

- **Step 2:** Choose an exercise (e.g., jumping squats, burpees, or mountain climbers) and perform it at maximum intensity for 20-30 seconds.

- **Step 3:** Rest for 10-15 seconds or perform a low-intensity exercise like marching in place during the rest period.

- **Step 4:** Repeat steps 2 and 3 for 4-5 cycles, gradually increasing the number of cycles as you progress.

- **Step 5:** Cool down with 5-10 minutes of stretching exercises to prevent muscle soreness.

3. Strength Training:

Strength training can involve various exercises and equipment. Here's a guide for a basic dumbbell workout:

- **Step 1:** Choose a set of dumbbells with an appropriate weight for your fitness level.

- **Step 2:** Perform compound exercises like squats, lunges, or deadlifts to work multiple muscle groups simultaneously.

- **Step 3:** Focus on proper form and technique to prevent injury. Consult a trainer or watch instructional videos if needed.

- **Step 4:** Perform 2-3 sets of each exercise, with 8-12 repetitions in each set.

- **Step 5:** Include exercises that target different muscle groups in your routine, such as bicep curls, tricep extensions, and shoulder presses.

- **Step 6:** Allow for adequate rest between sets to recover and prevent overexertion.

4. Running or Jogging:

Running or jogging is a simple yet effective exercise. Here's a basic guide:

- **Step 1:** Choose suitable running shoes and comfortable clothing.

- **Step 2:** Start with a warm-up by walking briskly or lightly jogging for 5-10 minutes.

- **Step 3:** Begin your run at a comfortable pace. Focus on your breathing and maintain good posture.

- **Step 4:** Gradually increase your pace or incorporate interval running (e.g., sprinting for 30 seconds and then jogging for 1-2 minutes).

- **Step 5:** Pay attention to your surroundings, enjoy the experience, and stay hydrated.

- **Step 6:** Cool down by walking for a few minutes to lower your heart rate and stretch your muscles.

5. Mindful Walking:

Mindful walking combines exercise with mindfulness. Here's a guide for a mindful walking practice:

- **Step 1:** Find a peaceful place for your walk, whether it's in nature or a quiet urban area.

- **Step 2:** Begin by standing still and taking a few deep breaths to center yourself.

- **Step 3:** Start walking at a slow, deliberate pace. Pay attention to each step, the sensation of your feet touching the ground, and your breath.

- **Step 4:** Engage your senses. Notice the sights, sounds, and smells around you without judgment.

- **Step 5:** If your mind starts to wander, gently bring your focus back to your walking and breathing.

- **Step 6:** Aim to walk for at least 10-15 minutes, gradually increasing the duration as you become more comfortable with the practice.

6. Cycling:

Cycling is a low-impact cardiovascular exercise. Here's how to get started:

- **Step 1:** Ensure you have a suitable bike in good condition, and wear a helmet for safety.

- **Step 2:** Begin with a warm-up by cycling at a moderate pace for 5-10 minutes.

- **Step 3:** Gradually increase your pace and resistance as you become comfortable.

- **Step 4:** Choose a route that matches your fitness level, whether it's a flat terrain for beginners or a challenging hill for more advanced cyclists.

- **Step 5:** Maintain good posture, keep your hands on the handlebars, and be mindful of traffic and road conditions.

- **Step 6:** Cool down by cycling at a slower pace for a few minutes and stretching your leg muscles.

7. Swimming:

Swimming is a full-body workout that's easy on the joints. Here's how to start:

- **Step 1:** Find a suitable swimming pool and wear appropriate swimwear.

- **Step 2:** Start with a warm-up by swimming at a slow pace for a few laps.

- **Step 3:** Choose your swimming style (e.g., freestyle, breaststroke, or backstroke) and swim at a comfortable pace.

- **Step 4:** Gradually increase the intensity and distance of your swim as your endurance improves.

- **Step 5:** Focus on proper technique and breathing while swimming.

- **Step 6:** Cool down by swimming at a slow pace for a few laps and stretching your muscles in the water.

8. Pilates:

Pilates is a low-impact exercise that focuses on core strength and flexibility. Here's a guide:

- **Step 1:** Find a Pilates class or use online resources for guided workouts.

- **Step 2:** Begin with a warm-up, which may include gentle stretches and breathing exercises.

- **Step 3:** Follow the instructor's guidance for various Pilates exercises that target different muscle groups.

- **Step 4:** Pay close attention to your form and breathing throughout the session.

- **Step 5:** Pilates exercises often involve controlled movements, so prioritize precision over speed.

- **Step 6:** Finish with a cool-down, which typically includes stretching and relaxation exercises.

9. Hiking:

Hiking is a great way to enjoy the outdoors while staying active. Here's how to prepare for a hike:

- **Step 1:** Choose a hiking trail that matches your fitness level and the time you have available.

- **Step 2:** Wear comfortable hiking boots or shoes and appropriate clothing for the weather.

- **Step 3:** Start your hike at a comfortable pace and gradually increase your speed as you go.

- **Step 4:** Stay hydrated by bringing water and snacks along.

- **Step 5:** Enjoy the scenery and take breaks to rest and appreciate nature.

- **Step 6:** After your hike, cool down by stretching your muscles and reflecting on your adventure.

10. Tai Chi:

Tai Chi is a gentle martial art that focuses on balance, flexibility, and relaxation. Here's how to practice Tai Chi:

- **Step 1:** Find a Tai Chi class or online tutorials to learn the movements.

- **Step 2:** Begin with a warm-up, which includes gentle stretches and deep breathing.

- **Step 3:** Follow the instructor's guidance for Tai Chi movements, which are slow and deliberate.

- **Step 4:** Pay attention to your posture, breathing, and the flow of your movements.

- **Step 5:** Tai Chi is often practiced in a meditative manner, promoting relaxation and mental clarity.

- **Step 6:** Conclude your session with deep breathing exercises and a sense of calm.

Conclusion:

You're not just a high-achiever; you're a high-potential, high-energy, high-dreamer who's destined for greatness. And the best part? Your body and mind are your most loyal allies on this journey. Treat them right, and they'll carry you to heights you've only dared to imagine.

So, here's to the high-octane you, fueled by the perfect blend of nutrition and exercise, racing towards your wildest dreams. Buckle up, because the world isn't ready for what you're about to achieve!

Until our next power-packed chat, keep soaring!

162

26 BEYOND THE BLUEPRINT: LIFELONG LEARNING AND ADAPTATION

Hello, perpetual learner!

You're like a sponge for knowledge, always thirsty for more. Lifelong learning isn't just a choice for you; it's a way of life. But why stop at what you already know? Let's embark on a journey that explores how continuous learning and adaptation can enrich your existence.

1. The Curious Mind: Why Lifelong Learning Matters

Curiosity didn't kill the cat; it's actually what keeps us alive and thriving. We'll dive into why feeding your inquisitive nature is like nectar for your soul.

2. Learning Beyond the Classroom: Everyday Lessons

Life itself is a classroom, and every experience, a lesson. We'll explore how to extract wisdom from even the most mundane moments.

3. The Digital Age: Leveraging Technology for Learning

In this tech-savvy world, knowledge is at your fingertips. Let's discuss how to harness the power of technology for your personal and professional growth.

4. Learning Styles: Finding What Works for You

Not all learners are created equal, and that's a good thing! Discover your unique learning style and tailor your approach to maximize retention and enjoyment.

5. Adapting to Change: The Art of Flexibility

Life doesn't follow a script, and sometimes, it throws curveballs. We'll delve into the art of adaptation and how a flexible mindset can be your secret weapon.

6. Mentors and Role Models: Learning from the Masters

Standing on the shoulders of giants isn't just a metaphor; it's a strategy for success. We'll discuss the importance of mentors and role models in your journey.

7. Reading as a Superpower

Reading isn't just a hobby; it's a superpower. We'll explore the benefits of reading and how it can transform your life.

8. The Joy of Unlearning

Sometimes, the path to growth involves unlearning what no longer serves you. We'll dive into the liberating concept of shedding old beliefs and habits.

9. Lifelong Learning in Practice: A Toolkit for Growth

Here, we'll equip you with practical strategies to incorporate continuous learning into your daily life, from setting learning goals to building a personal library.

The lifestyle patterns for various women's lifestyles with titles and key points:

1. Career-Oriented Professional:

Morning Routine:

- Wake up at 6:00 AM
- 10 minutes of mindfulness meditation
- 30 minutes of exercise (e.g., jogging or yoga)
- Nutritious breakfast

Work Hours:

- Busy work schedule with meetings and networking
- Short breaks for wellness activities
- Hydration and balanced lunch

Evening Routine:

- Return home, unwind, and have dinner
- Quality time with family or personal pursuits
- Relaxation and winding down

Weekends:

- Balance work and personal life
- Engage in hobbies and rest

2. Stay-at-Home Parent:

Morning Routine:

- Start the day early
- Prepare breakfast for the family
- Attend to children's needs and routines

Day Hours:

- Focus on childcare and household responsibilities
- Engage children in educational activities

Evening Routine:

- Family dinner and bonding time with children
- Relaxing activities

Weekends:

- Family outings and self-care
- Seek support from partners or relatives

3. Entrepreneur and Small Business Owner:

Morning Routine:

- Early start
- Meditation or goal-setting
- Work on business responsibilities

Work Hours:

- Manage business aspects, meetings, and planning
- Short breaks for well-being
- Healthy snacking habits

Evening Routine:

- Balance work with personal life
- Enjoy a balanced dinner
- Plan for the next day

Weekends:

- Business planning and networking
- Incorporate leisure activities

4. Fitness Enthusiast:

Morning Routine:

- Early start with vigorous workouts
- Nutritious, protein-rich breakfast

Work Hours:

- Fitness-related roles
- Recovery, nutrition planning, and relaxation

Weekends:

- Attend fitness classes or outdoor activities
- Plan fitness routines
- Incorporate relaxation

5. Student or Academic Professional:

Morning Routine:

- Attend classes, study, or research
- Varies based on academic schedule

Work Hours:

- Lectures, research, or administrative tasks
- Maintain work-life balance

Weekends:

- Catch up on assignments
- Engage in hobbies and relaxation

6. Creative Professional:

Morning Routine:

- Creative activities (e.g., writing, art, music)

Work Hours:

- Creative projects, meetings, or collaborations
- Attend artistic events and unwind

Weekends:

- Personal creativity and exploration

7. Retired or Senior Woman:

Morning Routine:

- Leisurely mornings
- Light exercises or hobbies
- Healthy breakfast

Day Hours:

- Pursue hobbies, socialize, or volunteer
- Enjoy relaxation and favorite activities

Weekends:

- Participate in senior community activities
- Explore local culture
- Maintain an active lifestyle

These lifestyle patterns highlight the titles and key points of daily routines for women with various roles and responsibilities.

Conclusion:

My dear lifelong learner, your journey is a tapestry of exploration, adaptation, and growth. With each new piece of knowledge, you're not just adding to your repertoire; you're evolving into the best version of yourself.

As you continue to embrace curiosity, adapt to change, and soak up wisdom from every source, remember that the journey itself is the destination. So, keep those synapses firing, those pages turning, and your heart open to the endless possibilities that lifelong learning brings.

Until our next chapter of discovery, keep exploring!

27 PREGNANCY PREP: NUTRITION AND LIFESTYLE FOR FERTILITY

Hey, beautiful future mamas!

Preparing for pregnancy is an exciting and significant step. It involves taking proactive steps to ensure your body is in the best possible shape to conceive and support a healthy pregnancy.

When we talk about nutrition for fertility, we're essentially talking about giving your body the right fuel for the journey ahead. Think of it as setting the stage for a healthy pregnancy. You want to focus on nutrient-rich foods that support reproductive health.

Folate is a big player here. It's crucial for preventing birth defects, so foods rich in folate, like leafy greens and citrus fruits, are a good addition to your diet. And don't forget healthy fats, like those found in fatty fish, flaxseeds, and walnuts. They can help maintain hormonal balance.

Protein is another important component, and it can be found in lean sources like chicken, beans, and tofu. Iron is vital too, so foods like red meat, beans, and leafy greens can help maintain proper levels.

Whole grains are great for complex carbohydrates and fiber, which support hormone regulation. And including plenty of antioxidant-rich foods, like fruits and vegetables, helps combat oxidative stress that can affect fertility.

Lifestyle plays a significant role in fertility as well. Achieving and maintaining a healthy weight is essential. Being either underweight or overweight can disrupt hormonal balance and affect your chances of conceiving.

Exercise is beneficial, but too much vigorous exercise can potentially impact fertility. It's all about finding the right balance that works for your body.

Stress management is vital too. High stress levels can throw hormones out of whack and affect ovulation. Incorporating relaxation techniques, whether it's yoga, meditation, or simply taking time for yourself, can be a game-changer.

Also, keep an eye on alcohol and caffeine intake. While moderate consumption is generally considered okay, excessive amounts can negatively affect fertility.

Lastly, if you smoke, quitting is highly advisable. Smoking has a detrimental impact on fertility for both men and women.

Some women may consider prenatal supplements, particularly those containing folic acid. These can be a valuable addition to your routine, but it's crucial to consult with a healthcare provider before starting any supplements to ensure they're right for your specific needs.

In essence, preparing for pregnancy is about taking a holistic approach to your health. Nutrition, lifestyle choices, and stress management all play crucial roles in optimizing fertility. Remember, each person's journey to conception is unique, so consulting with a healthcare provider is vital to address individual needs and concerns.

Whether you're just starting to think about expanding your family or you've been on this journey for a bit, let's chat about prepping for pregnancy. Because guess what? Pre-pregnancy health matters just as much as your health during pregnancy!

1. Fertility Overview: It's Not Just About the Baby Dance

Alright, before we jump into the nitty-gritty, let's set the stage. Fertility isn't just about the right timing; it's about creating the best possible environment for a baby to grow. Think of it like prepping soil before you plant a seed - the more nutrient-rich and well-tended it is, the better your plants (or in this case, babies) will grow!

2. The Nutrition-Fertility Link: It's Deeper Than You Think

You know how they say, "You are what you eat"? When it comes to fertility, this couldn't be more accurate. The food you consume can directly influence your reproductive health.

- **Macronutrients**: Carbs, fats, proteins. It's not just about quantity, but quality.

- **Micronutrients**: These are your vitamins and minerals. Essential for hormone regulation and egg quality.

3. The Superfoods for Super Moms-to-be

- **Leafy Greens**: Spinach, kale, and their friends are rich in folate, vital for preventing birth defects.

- **Full-Fat Dairy**: Some studies suggest that full-fat dairy can improve fertility. Maybe it's time to swap that skim milk for whole!

- **Oily Fish**: Salmon, mackerel, sardines are loaded with omega-3s. Great for hormone function and baby's brain development.

- **Complex Carbs**: Think quinoa, oats, and whole grains. They help stabilize your blood sugar, crucial for hormone balance.

- **Berries**: Loaded with antioxidants, they're perfect for protecting your eggs from damage.

4. Hydration Matters: Not Just H2O

It's not just about drinking 8 glasses of water. Hydration is key for cervical mucus (that stuff that helps sperm travel). Plus, consider herbal teas like raspberry leaf which can tone the uterus. But remember, moderation is key!

5. Exercise: Find Your Fertility Fit

Exercise is crucial, but there's a Goldilocks zone. Too little or too much can affect fertility.

- **Strength Training**: Great for muscle tone and overall health.

- **Yoga**: Especially fertility yoga, can be great for increasing blood flow to reproductive organs.

- **Cardio**: But not too much. Over-exercising can interfere with ovulation.

- **Walking**: Never underestimate a brisk 30-minute walk.

6. Weight: The Delicate Balance

Both extremes, underweight and overweight, can impact fertility. It's about balance and finding your body's happy medium.

7. The Caffeine & Alcohol Debate

- **Caffeine**: While an occasional cup of coffee is likely harmless, high caffeine intake might be linked to fertility issues.
- **Alcohol**: Moderate drinking probably won't hurt, but if you're actively trying, it might be best to cut back.

8. Stress: The Silent Fertility Feud

Chronic stress can mess with ovulation and even reduce libido. Time to embrace relaxation techniques:

- **Meditation**: Even 10 minutes a day can make a difference.
- **Deep Breathing**: Try the 4-7-8 technique.
- **Acupuncture**: Some women swear by it for fertility.

9. Supplements: Boosting Your Chances

- **Prenatal Vitamins**: Folic acid, iron, vitamin D, and calcium are top priorities.
- **Omega-3s**: If you're not a fish lover, consider a supplement.
- **CoQ10**: Some studies suggest it might improve egg quality.

(Always consult with a healthcare provider before starting any supplement!)

10. Ditching the Bad Habits

- **Smoking**: It's a big no-no. It can age your ovaries and deplete your eggs.

- **Recreational Drugs**: Best to avoid them. They can affect fertility and pose risks for a developing baby.

- **Over-the-counter meds**: Some can interfere with fertility. Always chat with your doc.

11. The Male Factor: It Takes Two to Tango

While we're focusing on the ladies, remember, male fertility matters too! Encourage your partner to adopt a healthy lifestyle, limit alcohol, and consider a multivitamin.

Wrap-Up: Your Body, Your Journey

Prepping for pregnancy is a journey, not a destination. Everyone's path to motherhood is unique, so remember to be patient with yourself. Celebrate the small victories and know that with every nutritious bite, every rejuvenating exercise, and every stress-reducing breath, you're taking a step closer to welcoming a new life. Here's to you and your journey to motherhood. You've got this, mama-to-be!

Whew! That was quite a ride, right? But always remember that every body is different. What works wonders for one might not work for another. Stay in tune with yourself, and always, always consult with a healthcare professional on your fertility journey.

28 MOVING THROUGH MOTHERHOOD: EXERCISE DURING AND POST-PREGNANCY

Hey, radiant mama!

Exercise plays a crucial role in a woman's journey through motherhood, both during and after pregnancy. It's about nurturing your body and ensuring your well-being, as well as setting a positive example for your child.

During pregnancy, exercise can provide a multitude of benefits. It helps improve mood, reduces the risk of excessive weight gain, and supports overall physical health. Gentle activities like walking, swimming, and prenatal yoga can be especially beneficial. These exercises help with circulation, ease back pain, and prepare your body for labor.

However, it's essential to consult with your healthcare provider before beginning or continuing an exercise routine during pregnancy. They can provide guidance on the most suitable activities based on your individual health and any potential complications.

After giving birth, exercise can be a fantastic way to aid recovery and regain strength. It can help improve posture, increase energy levels, and enhance overall well-being during what can be a challenging time.

Engaging in postpartum exercises that target the core and pelvic floor muscles is particularly valuable. These muscles may be weakened during pregnancy and childbirth, and specific exercises can help in their recovery. Activities like postpartum yoga or Pilates can be excellent choices.

It's crucial to listen to your body during the postpartum period. Every woman's experience is unique, and it's essential not to rush into strenuous exercise. Start gradually, and don't hesitate to seek guidance from a postpartum fitness specialist or physical therapist.

Remember, postpartum exercise is not just about returning to your pre-pregnancy shape; it's about building strength, boosting energy, and promoting emotional well-being during this transformative period.

Finding time for exercise as a new mother can be a challenge, but it's essential to prioritize self-care. Incorporate your baby into your routine if needed; activities like stroller walks or mom-and-baby yoga classes can be enjoyable bonding experiences.

Additionally, consider enlisting support from friends and family to allow you some time for self-care, including exercise. Your health and well-being are essential not only for you but for your child as well.

So, you're journeying through the incredible path of motherhood. From the fluttery first kicks to the post-baby belly laughs, this is undoubtedly one of the most transformational times in a woman's life. And guess what? Your body is doing some genuinely superhero-level stuff right now. With that in mind, let's chat about moving that wonderful body of yours during and after pregnancy, shall we?

1. First Things First: Why Exercise?

You might be wondering, "Why bother with squats when there's a nursery to decorate?" Well, exercise during pregnancy is like giving your body a super boost. It helps manage weight gain, boosts mood, improves sleep, and can even ease those pesky aches and pains. Post-pregnancy, it aids in recovery and helps you keep up with your ever-active little one.

2. Embracing Changes: Your Body's New Normal

Girl, pregnancy is a whirlwind of change! As your bump grows, your center of gravity shifts. Your joints loosen thanks to a hormone called relaxin. And let's not even start on the mammary metamorphosis! All these changes mean that the exercises you were doing pre-pregnancy might need some tweaking.

3. First Trimester: Setting the Stage

Those first 12 weeks can be a rollercoaster. Morning sickness, anyone? But if you're up for it:

- **Cardio**: Low impact stuff like walking or swimming can be great.

- **Strength Training**: Focus on light weights and more reps.

- **Yoga**: Opt for prenatal classes. They're tailored for mamas-to-be.

And always, always listen to your body. If you're not feeling it, it's okay to take a break!

4. Second Trimester: The Golden Period

For many mamas, this is the sweet spot. Morning sickness usually eases up, and energy levels might be higher.

- **Pelvic Floor Exercises**: These are GOLD. They'll help with delivery and recovery.

- **Low-Impact Aerobics**: Think dance or aqua aerobics.

- **Pilates**: It's great for core strength, but be mindful of the moves.

Remember, lying flat on your back is a no-no now because it can reduce blood flow to your baby.

5. Third Trimester: Navigating the Home Stretch

Oh boy (or girl!), things are getting real now. Your bump's bigger, and you might feel more tired.

- **Walking**: Simple and effective.

- **Stretching**: Helps with muscle tension.

- **Pelvic Tilts**: Great for back pain.

Avoid exercises that risk any abdominal trauma or strain.

6. Postpartum: The Fourth Trimester

Baby's here! Now, it's a mix of joy, exhaustion, and perhaps a longing to feel like 'yourself' again.

- **Start Slow**: Your body just did an amazing thing. Give it time to heal.

- **Walking**: Start with short strolls and gradually increase.

- **Postnatal Yoga**: Tailored for post-baby bodies, it's gentle and restorative.

7. Diastasis Recti: Mind the Gap

This sounds fancy, but it's just a separation between your abdominal muscles. It's common post-pregnancy. If you've got it, certain exercises can help, while others can exacerbate it. Always check with a physiotherapist or specialist.

8. Breastfeeding and Exercise

Good news! Moderate exercise doesn't affect milk production or quality. Just ensure you're consuming enough calories and staying hydrated. A supportive bra is a must!

9. Emotional Well-being: It's Not Just Physical

Postpartum emotions are a wild ride. Exercise can help boost mood, thanks to those lovely endorphins. If you're feeling blue or overwhelmed, always reach out. You're not alone, mama.

10. C-Section Mamas: Your Unique Journey

A C-section is major surgery. Recovery takes time, and exercise post-surgery is a whole different ball game. Always follow your doctor's advice on when and how to start.

11. Listening to Your Body

This bears repeating. Always, ALWAYS, listen to your body. If something doesn't feel right, stop. You know your body best.

Wrap Up: Embrace Your Pace

Whether you're a seasoned gym bunny or someone who's just dipping their toes into the world of fitness, remember: every body and every pregnancy is different. Celebrate the small victories, cherish this unique journey, and always prioritize your well-being.

To the ever-evolving, ever-amazing journey of motherhood, here's to moving with purpose, joy, and embracing every beautiful change along the way. You're doing great, mama.

Whew! That's a wrap for this chapter. Remember, while it's great to gather info and advice, your healthcare provider's guidance is crucial. Always consult them about your exercise regimen during and post-pregnancy. Until next time!

29 NURTURING NUTRITION IN PREGNANCY: EATING FOR TWO

Hey there, glowing goddess! 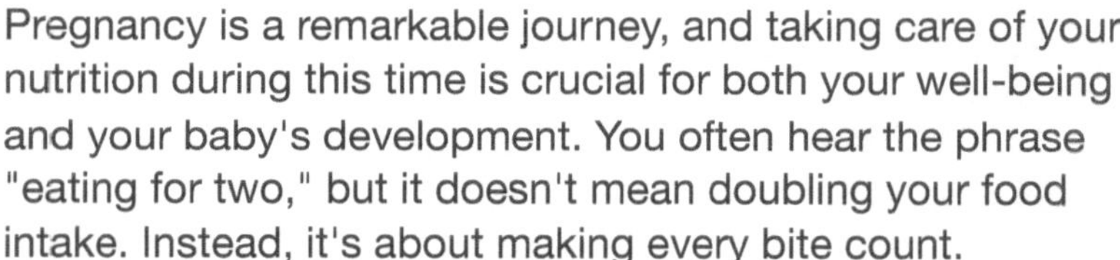

Pregnancy is a remarkable journey, and taking care of your nutrition during this time is crucial for both your well-being and your baby's development. You often hear the phrase "eating for two," but it doesn't mean doubling your food intake. Instead, it's about making every bite count.

Your body goes through significant changes during pregnancy, and your nutritional needs change accordingly. The goal is to provide all the essential nutrients to support your baby's growth and development. A well-balanced diet is your ally here, ensuring you get a wide range of vital nutrients.

Protein, for instance, is essential because it helps develop your baby's organs and tissues. Think about including lean protein sources like poultry, fish, beans, and tofu in your meals.

Folate is another superstar nutrient during pregnancy. It's crucial for preventing neural tube defects in your baby. You can find folate in foods like leafy greens, citrus fruits, and fortified cereals. Many women also take prenatal vitamins containing folic acid, the synthetic form of folate.

Calcium is necessary for your baby's bones and teeth, so be sure to include dairy products, fortified plant-based milk, and leafy greens in your diet.

Iron plays a role in preventing anemia during pregnancy. You can source iron from red meat, poultry, beans, and leafy greens. Pairing iron-rich foods with those rich in vitamin C can enhance absorption.

Fiber is your friend for digestion and preventing constipation, a common pregnancy woe. Whole grains, fruits, and vegetables are fiber-rich options.

Staying well-hydrated is essential too. Water supports your increased blood volume needs during pregnancy and helps prevent dehydration.

While it's true that you need extra calories during pregnancy, it's not an excuse to go overboard. Instead, focus on nutrient-dense foods that provide all those essential vitamins and minerals without excessive calories.

It's crucial to remember that every pregnancy is unique. Factors like your age, activity level, and any existing health conditions can affect your nutritional needs. That's why working closely with your healthcare provider is essential. They can create a personalized nutrition plan that suits your unique needs and ensures a healthy pregnancy for both you and your baby.

So, you've embarked on this wondrous journey of pregnancy. Suddenly, you're not just feeding yourself – there's a tiny human in there depending on you too. The old adage says, "You're eating for two." But what does that *really* mean? Grab a comfy seat (and maybe a snack), and let's dive deep into the world of nurturing nutrition during pregnancy.

1. Myth-Busting Time: "Eating for Two"

Alright, let's get this straight: "Eating for two" doesn't mean doubling your food intake. Bummer, I know! Instead, it's about nourishing both you and your baby optimally. Think quality over quantity.

2. Caloric Needs: The Nitty Gritty

During your first trimester, you don't actually need extra calories. Yep, you read that right! In the second trimester, an additional 340 calories a day should do, and by the third, about 450 extra calories. It's not as much as you'd think, but it's all about *nutrient-rich* calories.

3. Protein Power

Protein's the building block of life. Especially crucial now, for both baby's growth and to support your expanding blood volume, breasts, and uterus.

- **Great sources**: Lean meats, poultry, fish, tofu, legumes, eggs, and nuts.

- **Tip**: Fish is fabulous, but avoid high-mercury ones like shark, swordfish, and mackerel. Aim for safer options like salmon, shrimp, or catfish.

4. Carb Talk: Fueling Up

Not all carbs are created equal. Let's aim for the good stuff, alright?

- **Whole Grains**: Think brown rice, quinoa, and oats.

- **Fruits and Veggies**: Oh, the colorful bounty! Berries, oranges, leafy greens – they're all packed with essential nutrients.

5. Fats: The Good, the Bad, the Ugly

Fats are crucial for baby's brain development and for absorbing certain vitamins. But, as with carbs, choose wisely.

- **Fantastic Fats**: Avocados, nuts, seeds, and olive oil.

- **Fats to Limit**: Saturated and trans fats, like those in deep-fried foods.

6. Don't Forget Fiber!

Trust me on this: with the pregnancy hormones and your growing uterus, constipation can become a *thing*. Fiber is your bestie here.

- **Fab sources**: Whole grains, fruits, veggies, and legumes.

7. Calcium for Strong Bones

Both you and your baby need this for strong bones and teeth. Plus, it helps your circulatory, muscular, and nervous systems run smoothly.

- **Dairy Delights**: Milk, yogurt, cheese.

- **Dairy-Free**: Almonds, leafy greens, fortified foods, and seeds.

8. Iron: Keep the Energy Flowing

Your blood volume is increasing to support your baby, and you need iron to make hemoglobin for all that extra blood.

- **Iron-rich foods**: Lean meats, poultry, fish, tofu, beans, and iron-fortified cereals.

9. Folic Acid: The BFF of Early Pregnancy

Crucial in the early stages to prevent neural tube defects.

- **Fantastic Foods**: Leafy greens, fortified cereals, legumes, and citrus fruits.

10. Stay Hydrated, Mama!

Water plays a vital role in forming the placenta and amniotic fluid. Keep that water bottle handy and sip throughout the day.

11. Limiting Caffeine and Sugar

I know, I know – who doesn't love a latte or a sweet treat? But let's try to limit them for now. Excess caffeine and sugar can lead to unwanted complications.

12. Listen to Your Cravings (Within Reason)

Pickles at midnight? Chocolate-covered strawberries? Our bodies sometimes tell us what they need through cravings. But always pair them with some common sense.

13. Foods to Approach with Caution

Sorry to be a party pooper, but some foods carry risks during pregnancy:

- **Raw seafood**: Like sushi.

- **Unpasteurized foods**: Think soft cheeses.

- **High-mercury fish**: As mentioned earlier.

- **Raw eggs**: Sorry, cookie dough lovers!

14. Vitamins & Supplements

It can be tough to get all the nutrients you need from food alone. Prenatal vitamins can help bridge the gap, but always discuss with your healthcare provider.

15. Nausea & Heartburn: The Unwanted Guests

Morning sickness can be a misnomer – it can strike at any time. Small, frequent meals and snacks like crackers can help. As for heartburn, eating slowly, avoiding spicy and acidic foods, and not lying down right after eating can be beneficial.

16. Cultivate a Positive Relationship with Food

Remember, mama, nourishing your body is an act of love – for both you and your baby. Celebrate this time, enjoy your meals, and trust that you're doing your best.

Phew! That was quite the food journey, wasn't it? You're equipped with some solid knowledge now. But remember, every pregnancy is unique. It's always a good idea to work with a nutritionist or healthcare provider to tailor things to your needs.

Stay nourished, keep glowing, and until next time – happy eating!

30 CONCLUSION: YOUR THRIVING JOURNEY – MOVING FORWARD WITH CONFIDENCE AND GRACE

Congratulations, radiant soul!

You've embarked on a journey through the intricacies of female health, wellness, and empowerment. From understanding the marvels of your body to discovering the power of nourishing food, exercise, and mindful living, you've delved deep into the beautiful tapestry that is the female experience.

As you stand here at the conclusion of our voyage, take a moment to reflect on the path you've traveled. You've absorbed wisdom about nutrition, exercise, mental well-being, and the importance of lifelong learning. You've explored the intricate dance of hormones, discovered the art of self-care, and recognized the significance of social connections.

But remember, dear reader, this journey doesn't end here; it merely transforms. Armed with knowledge, inspiration, and a renewed sense of self, you're now equipped to embrace your uniqueness and navigate the ever-evolving terrain of your life with confidence and grace.

Here are a few key takeaways to carry with you:

- **Self-Care is Not Selfishness:** Prioritize self-care without guilt. It's the foundation upon which your well-being and happiness are built.

- **Embrace Your Body:** Your body is not your enemy; it's your lifelong companion. Love, honor, and respect it for the incredible vessel it is.

- **Nutrition is Your Ally:** Food is not just fuel; it's medicine. Choose your sustenance wisely, and it will support you in countless ways.

- **Exercise is Empowerment:** Movement isn't a punishment; it's a celebration of your strength and vitality. Find joy in it.

- **Mindfulness is a Superpower:** Your mental and emotional well-being are equally important as your physical health. Nurture your mind and heart.

- **Connection is Nourishment:** Cultivate meaningful relationships. Your tribe is your source of strength and support.

- **Never Stop Learning:** Curiosity is your compass. Keep exploring, adapting, and growing.

- **You Are Your Own Blueprint:** While you've gathered insights and knowledge from these pages, remember that your unique journey is yours to craft. You are the author of your story, the architect of your health, and the curator of your happiness.

So, my dear, as you close this chapter and begin the next, may you carry the wisdom, strength, and inspiration gained from our journey together. You are a force of nature, a beacon of resilience, and a symbol of possibility.

With confidence and grace, move forward on your path of thriving. Embrace each day as a new opportunity to celebrate the incredible woman you are.

Until we meet again, dear friend, keep eating, moving, and thriving. Your journey has only just begun.

With boundless love and admiration,

Kiran Vekariya

ABOUT THE AUTHOR

Kiran Vekariya's story is nothing short of remarkable. She had a vision - a vision to make the world a healthier and fitter place. But here's the twist: she embarked on this mission during a time when she herself was facing a storm of challenges. Picture this - financial struggles, an identity crisis, and the daunting world of fitness, which is incredibly competitive. It was a tough road, but Kiran's determination to make a positive impact on the world's health was unwavering.

So, what did she do? She started her own fitness studio, which she aptly named KFS, in eastern Ahmedabad, Gujarat. But this wasn't just about workouts and diets; it was about holistic well-being. Kiran realized that true fitness goes beyond physicality. It's about mental and social health too. She understood that you can't be truly fit without addressing personal issues, both physical and emotional.

Kiran started helping women with their personal challenges, diseases, and social well-being. For men, it was about mental fitness, financial stability, and soft skills, not just building muscles. Her scientific approach and empathy-driven guidance started yielding amazing results. Her clients weren't just getting physically fit; they were experiencing positive changes in their mental health too. She became not just a fitness instructor but a life mentor.

One of her clients, Remy, was so inspired by Kiran's mission that he left his real estate business to join her. Together, they were making a real impact on people's lives. But then, like a plot twist in a movie, the pandemic hit. It hit hard, and Kiran's business suffered. But here's the incredible part - she didn't abandon her clients. She refunded their fees and continued helping them for free. This was more than a business; it was a mission.

When the pandemic storm calmed down, Kiran's finances were in ruins. But she didn't give up. With Remy's support, she started a new fitness studio in a different location, and her loyal clients flocked to her. Just when things were looking up, Kiran faced another life-altering challenge - a cancer diagnosis. Her dream of helping countless people attain better health seemed in jeopardy.

But Kiran didn't back down. With unwavering determination, she not only defeated cancer but also made a remarkable recovery in just 40 days. She emerged stronger and healthier than ever, ready to take her mission to even greater heights.

Kiran's response to adversity was to expand KFS's offerings. She introduced a corporate wing, franchising options, personalized courses, and even a fitness and wellness institute. Today, KFS stands as a testament to Kiran's resilience and her unwavering dedication to the well-being of others. It's become the fastest-growing fitness and wellness company in India, touching the lives of over 12,800 individuals and curing countless diseases.

Kiran Vekariya's story is a testament to the power of determination, resilience, and the unwavering commitment to wellness. Her journey from facing adversity to triumph is an inspiration to all of us, reminding us that no matter how tough the road may seem, with passion and a commitment to health, we can achieve incredible transformations.

KFS's mission is simple yet profound: to provide holistic fitness, including physical, mental, and social well-being, to everyone. Kiran's legacy is a shining beacon of hope, proving that with determination and a deep-rooted commitment to well-being, we can achieve remarkable transformations.

NOTE

NOTE

NOTE

NOTE

NOTE